ALSO BY ARTHUR LAZARUS

Neuroleptic Malignant Syndrome and Related Conditions (co-author)

Controversies in Managed Mental Health Care

Career Pathways in Psychiatry: Transition in Changing Times

MD/MBA: Physicians on the New Frontier of Medical Management

*Every Story Counts: Examining Contemporary
Practice Through Narrative Medicine*

MEDICINE ON FIRE

A NARRATIVE TRAVELOGUE

ARTHUR LAZARUS, MD, MBA

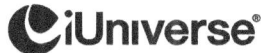

MEDICINE ON FIRE
A NARRATIVE TRAVELOGUE

iUniverse books may be ordered through booksellers or by contacting:

iUniverse
1663 Liberty Drive
Bloomington, IN 47403
www.iuniverse.com
844-349-9409

Because of the dynamic nature of the Internet, any web addresses or links contained in this book may have changed since publication and may no longer be valid. The views expressed in this work are solely those of the author and do not necessarily reflect the views of the publisher, and the publisher hereby disclaims any responsibility for them.

Any people depicted in stock imagery provided by Getty Images are models, and such images are being used for illustrative purposes only. Certain stock imagery © Getty Images.

ISBN: 978-1-6632-5727-7 (sc)
ISBN: 978-1-6632-5728-4 (e)

Library of Congress Control Number: 2023920303

Print information available on the last page.

iUniverse rev. date: 01/10/2024

Dedicated to the memory of my parents,
Aaron and Lenore Lazarus.
May their flame burn bright, always.

Contents

About the Author

Arthur L. Lazarus, MD, MBA, is a healthcare consultant, certified physician executive, and nationally recognized author, speaker, and champion of physician leadership and wellness. He has broad experience in clinical practice and the health insurance industry, having led programs at Cigna and Humana. At Humana, Lazarus was vice president and corporate medical director of behavioral health operations in Louisville, Kentucky, and subsequently a population health medical director for the state of Florida.

Lazarus has also held leadership positions in several pharmaceutical companies, including Pfizer and AstraZeneca, conducting clinical trials, and reviewing promotional material for medical accuracy and FDA compliance. He has published more than 250 articles in scientific and professional journals and has written five books, including *Neuroleptic Malignant Syndrome and Related Conditions, Controversies in Managed Mental Health Care, Career Pathways in Psychiatry, MD/MBA: Physicians on the New Frontier of Medical Management,* and *Every Story Counts: Exploring Contemporary Practice Through Narrative Medicine.*

Born in Philadelphia, Pennsylvania, Lazarus attended Boston University, where he graduated with a bachelor's degree in psychology with Distinction. He received his medical degree with Honors from Temple University School of Medicine, followed by a psychiatric residency at Temple University Hospital, where he was chief resident. After residency, Lazarus joined the faculty of Temple University School of Medicine, where he currently serves as adjunct professor of Psychiatry. He also holds non-faculty appointments as Executive-in-Residence at

Temple University Fox School of Business and Management, where he received his MBA degree, and Senior Fellow, Jefferson College of Population Health, Philadelphia, Pennsylvania.

Well known for his leadership and medical management skills, Lazarus is a sought-after presenter, mentor, teacher, and writer. He has shared his expertise and perspective at numerous local, national, and international meetings and seminars.

Lazarus is a past president of the American Association for Psychiatric Administration and Leadership, a former member of the board of directors of the American Association for Physician Leadership (AAPL), and a current member of the AAPL editorial review board. In 2010, the American Psychiatric Association honored Lazarus with the Administrative Psychiatry Award for his effectiveness as an administrator of major mental health programs and expanding the body of knowledge of management science in mental health services delivery systems.

Lazarus is among a select group of physicians in the United States who have been inducted into both the Alpha Omega Alpha medical honor society and the Beta Gamma Sigma honor society of collegiate schools of business.

Lazarus lives with his wife near Charlotte, North Carolina. They have four adult children. He enjoys walking, biking, playing piano, and listening to music.

"The practice of medicine is an art, not a trade;
a calling, not a business; a calling in which your heart
will be exercised equally with your head."
—Sir William Osler

Preface

Singer-songwriter David Byrne (Talking Heads) asked: "Say something once, why say it again?" To which I rejoin: Write a book about narrative medicine, why write another one?

This is my second book of narrative essays, coming quickly on the heels of my first collection: *Every Story Counts: Exploring Contemporary Practice Through Narrative Medicine*. The answer to Byrne's question – why say something again? – is because the impulse to write never ceases. It may fade and sometimes extinguish like a fire, but narrative impulses are hard-wired into our brains and are basic to our being. That's why I decided to title this collection of essays *Medicine on Fire: A Narrative Travelogue*, because the narrative burns in every one of us, and because the field of narrative medicine is hot and on fire right now.

The "travelogue" relates to my experience as a student in a formal university-based narrative medicine program, never imagining that I would find myself wandering through the virtual halls of graduate school nearing my eighth decade, sharing stories with much younger classmates and writing narratives flavored with memoir, many included in this book.

In "Memory and Imagination," Patricia Hampl writes: "Memoir is travel writing," with the memoirist moving through mountains, deserts, and green places – "moving through it all faithfully, not so much a survivor with a harrowing tale to tell as that older sort of traveler, the pilgrim, seeking, wondering." Indeed, our most ancient metaphor says life is a journey.

I paused my journey soon after I punctuated and proofread the final essay in *Every Story Counts*. I began to write again not least because there was more storytelling left in me, yet I was careful not to repeat my stories. Also, the stakes were much different writing as a student. I was paying more attention to the craft of writing and to my audience – ostensibly other students, but also those who might be my critics. What did they think of my writing skills? How well did *they* write? What topics did they choose to write about. Did I measure up? Flashbacks to medical school? You bet!

Fortunately, our writing instructor established a "no stress policy." In our syllabus accompanying "Introduction to Narrative Medicine," she wrote: "Begin the day with quiet for yourself rather than stress and panic. We all have PTSD right now from the pandemic and other insurmountable forces. So, begin the day with peace and carry it with you for as long as you can." She continued – and this was the best part – "Regarding coursework, getting stressed about creativity is like getting stressed about yoga. Don't. Sit down with laptop, phone, pen, paper. Do this as often as possible. It only takes two minutes to get some words out. If something starts to flow, stay with it. If nothing does, that's okay. No stress."

My Yoda-like instructor spoke as she wrote: softy and reassuringly, with an ethereal quality. "You are all welcome here, and all of you is welcome," she repeatedly told our class. My teacher reminded me of a cherished professor, one who told our medical school class during orientation that "we all belong here."

Now it is my turn to extend a warm and welcoming invitation to you, not only as a reader, but also as a writer, perhaps an active writer, or a latent one like me. As we venture forward, I will be your guide, your humble shepherd and storyteller. We will explore narrative medicine in its many forms – knowledge, training, practice, illness, and healing – and in the process uncover profound intuitions about the therapeutic benefits of the narrative.

We will be able to grasp the essence of narrative medicine, which, according to Lewis Mehl-Madrona, MD, PhD, one of the pioneers of the narrative medicine movement, is appreciating the rich stories we have gained in our training, those brought to us by our patients and their families, while "seeing ourselves as coauthors in the creation of new stories that have uncertain endings, at least while they are being written."

Our journey will definitely have an ending, and I guarantee it will be memorable.

NARRATIVE AS A FORM
OF KNOWLEDGE

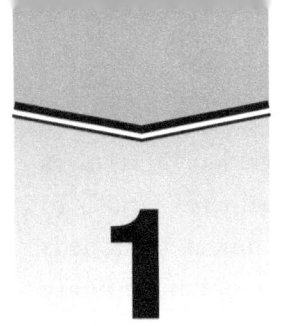

Transitioning from Academic Writing to the Narrative

An alternative writing style can give a voice to our patients' stories.

Many doctors feel that writing is a struggle. "They delay. They feel inadequate – even inauthentic," wrote psychiatrists Laura Weiss Roberts, MD, MA, and John Coverdale MD, MEd, who are editor-in-chief and associate editor, respectively, of *Academic Medicine*. Roberts and Coverdale continue: "While these colleagues may view teaching and healing as natural capacities, they view writing as anything but."

"How should I write?" I asked a mentor when I was a medical resident. He replied, "Art, just write what you want to say." Indeed, a fellow student in my narrative medicine writing class reminded me that the definition of a writer is "someone who writes."

Still, there has been a slight hitch – I wasn't trained in the narrative. My mentor was a well-published physician researcher trained in the scientific method, and that's how I learned to write – scientifically and technically, without jargon, adhering to the no nonsense "instructions for authors" in the likes of *JAMA* and its sister specialty journals. (To their credit, *JAMA* and other major medical journals now consider narratives and poetry for publication.)

Academic writing primarily focuses on the objective presentation of facts and data in a structured, formal manner. Its emphasis on empirical evidence, research, and statistical data is often used to advance medical science and share new knowledge. It involves a clear, concise, and formal style of writing that adheres strictly to specific formats and standards. The language is technical, the tone is impersonal, the expectation is precision and accuracy, and the primary goal is to inform, educate, and persuade based on facts and figures.

In contrast, narrative medicine writing is a form of reflective writing that centers on the experiences of patients and clinicians. It utilizes storytelling to explore the emotional, psychological, and social aspects of healthcare. The language is more personal, descriptive, and emotive, focusing on the human experience rather than just the clinical facts. The goal is to foster empathy, compassion, and a deeper understanding of the patient's perspective, thereby enhancing patient care and the overall healthcare experience.

Doctors often find their inspiration in narrative medicine because the discipline guides them in the art of empathic listening and allows them to be more responsive to their patients' needs. Medical training has the opposite effect. Openness and beneficence are suppressed by conditioning, forcing students to sacrifice compassion in the name of intellectual clarity. Declaring that physicians must remain dispassionate and detached from their emotions to ensure patient care is anathema to narrative practice.

I have had to unlearn the academic way of thinking and writing to write narratively. In doing so, there is a risk that I will be viewed as a heretic by my colleagues, or at least labeled as a "breezy" writer. Sometimes I feel like an outcast depicted in a surreal scene in the *Field of Dreams*, where Terence Mann (James Earl Jones) sprays Ray Kinsella (Kevin Costner) with an insecticide mist, exclaiming, "Out! Back to the sixties! Back! There's no place for you here in the future!" You could substitute "academia" for "the future" and understand my predicament.

So, how am I finding my writer's voice? Or, to paraphrase John Fox, the author of *Poetic Medicine*, am I finding yeast in my words so that my prose will become like "fresh bread on the table," leavened with experience, resilience and intuitive understanding? I'll answer in a moment, but first let me tell you about Fox.

Fox is an educator and a certified poetry therapist who believes he has been "called" to poetry as a form of healing. He claims that poetry is a "natural medicine." Fox likes the feeling-oriented, non-linear logic of poetry because it allows for paradox and even celebrates it. After all, isn't the presence of paradox ubiquitous in medicine: joy and woe; pain and comfort; sadness and exaltation?

Unfortunately, the poetry of my youth has left a sour taste that I cannot cleanse. In the preface to Fox's book, the *New York Times* best-selling physician author Rachel Naomi Remen, MD, observes: "Much of the old poetry was pretentious and erudite, full of references to mythology or the ancient Greeks, poetry whose words I could not easily understand." My sentiment exactly!

I understand that modern poetry is different. Nevertheless, I have turned to other sources and forms of writing to help me unleash my inner self on paper, specifically to break free from an academic climate that is increasingly insular, and often reflects the narrow-minded vision of clinical investigators, grant-writers and pseudo-scientific scholars. I am breaking free of those literary gatekeepers by reading essays written by physicians and non-physician authors from multicultural perspectives and backgrounds: Black, Latino, Indigenous, Asian, Middle Eastern, LGBTQ+ – or a combination of those identities – and by participating in writing exercises.

The multicultural writers have reminded me that institutions, particularly academic centers with their strict rules, formats, and expectations, can feel stifling and limit individual expression, in essence impeding learning by teaching exclusively to scientific analyses and objective understandings, neglecting the creative, spiritual and cognitive dimensions underlying practice.

Stated differently by Kandace Creel Falcón while pursuing her doctorate degree as a Xicana femme feminist: "The PhD track is supposed to discipline you. During my time as a graduate student

3

the process tried to beat me out of my writing...Soon I could no longer recognize myself in my pages. I had been disciplined." Falcón's personal battle was to push against the forces of the academy that sought to minimize and invalidate her perspective. Her triumph over academic tyranny prevented her from becoming lost in her own stories.

I, too, believe that breaking free of the academic gatekeepers is the first – and most important – step in bridging the gap between academic writing and narrative medicine writing. Once unchained, other steps considered prerequisite for narrative writing seem to quickly follow:

- Adopting a mindset that values the patient's story as much as the clinical data.
- Listening deeply and empathically to capture the nuances of the patient's experiences.
- Weaving the patients' experiences – hope, fears, emotions, and aspirations – into a coherent, engaging narrative that captures the reader's attention and evokes empathy.
- Employing narrative techniques such as scene-setting, character development, and plot construction; and
- Using language that is accessible and relatable to a broad audience.

The transition from academic writing to narrative medicine writing is a challenging but rewarding journey that requires a profound and fundamental change in mindset, approach, and style. Making the transition requires a commitment to use writing as a tool to enhance healthcare by finding a voice and giving voice to our patients' stories.

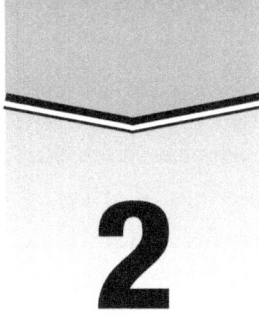

2

For Whom the Narrative Tolls

Pay attention to your writing audience, and cast a wide net.

Soon after the preceding essay appeared online in *MedPage Today* (September 19, 2023), a reader commented: "Very interesting and on target for this ancient, retired academic. But the intended audience for these narratives is not clear to me."

I never gave much thought about my "audience." I write on a whim, when I'm moved to do so. I don't write for a living. I'm not forced to "publish or perish." I don't have an agent. I just write about what appeals to me and hope some website or book publisher will think it is worthy of dissemination online or in print. I think that's how many physicians approach writing – from the heart, often about frustration with the health system – and they write for many of the same reasons patients write: stress relief, self-care, and sharing experiences. Exceptions include the elite physician writers who have agents and best-selling books to their credit, although their reasons for writing do not seem much different than the typical physician in practice.

The more I thought about the comment from the "retired academic," the more I realized that all writers, from amateurs like me to the most dedicated and professional among us, should have an audience in mind before writing and know something about that audience. So, I divided the academic's comment into two questions. First, **who is the intended audience for narratives written by patients?** Second, **who is the**

intended audience for narratives written by healthcare practitioners? Of course, the two groups – patients and practitioners – are not mutually exclusive, and their reasons for writing do indeed overlap.

The intended audience for narratives written by patients can be diverse. It includes healthcare providers like physicians, nurses, and other medical professionals who need to understand the patient's story for better diagnosis and treatment. It can also be intended for patients and their families to help them understand the disease and its impacts. Additionally, it could be for medical students and researchers studying specific cases, or even policy makers who can use these narratives to inform healthcare policies.

The intended audience for narratives written by healthcare practitioners may be more wide ranging. Readers include:

1. **Other healthcare professionals**: These narratives can help in sharing knowledge, experience, and best practices among peers.
2. **Patients and their families**: Healthcare professionals sometimes write narratives to explain complex medical conditions and procedures in a way that is easier for patients and their families to understand.
3. **Medical students and trainees**: Narratives can be used as teaching tools to illustrate real-life clinical scenarios and ethical dilemmas.
4. **Researchers and academics**: Narratives can provide valuable insights into patient experiences and outcomes for research purposes.
5. **Administrators and policy makers**: These narratives can help illustrate the impact of certain policies or lack thereof, guiding decisions in healthcare management, policy development and the law.
6. **The general public**: Some narratives are intended to educate the general public about health issues, promote public health, or advocate for certain health policy positions.

Whenever I think about the writer's audience, whether written from the perspective of a patient or provider, I'm reminded of the well-known phrase: "Never send to know for whom the bell tolls; it tolls for thee," which originates in one of John Donne's most famous pieces of prose writing: *Devotions Upon Emergent Occasions, Meditation XVII.*

"No man is an island, entire of itself; every man is a piece of the continent, a part of the main; if a clod be washed away by the sea, Europe is the less, as well as if a promontory were, as well as if a manor of thy friend's or of thine own were; any man's death diminishes me, because I am involved in mankind, and therefore *never send to know for whom the bell tolls; it tolls for thee* [italics added]."

Donne's *Meditations* concern man's spiritual and social well-being, especially with regard to illness and death. Donne was close to death when he wrote that passage, in itself a form of narrative medicine writing. He was exploring man's interconnectedness and saying we are all one and that, when someone dies, a piece of us dies with that person. I fashion it to the "circle of life" ideology based on the belief that every living thing exists as part of a delicate balance in nature, a series of events that unfolds on earth, bringing us from cradle to grave, through ups and downs, love and misfortune, and so on.

It is understandable that we should feel a sense of belonging to all things in life and, along with it, a sense of loss at every death, because dying diminishes the ranks of humankind and potential contributions by those no longer with us. The other famous phrase from this reflective paragraph that has entered the vernacular is "no man is an island," because no individual can subsist alone. Donne foreshadowed the epidemic of loneliness that exists today.

Writing that stems from healers and patients begs for social awareness and connectivity. Narrative writers desire companionship and community, a means to share their feelings and let their feelings be known. It's trite to say, but we all belong to one race – the human race – and all of us are affected by suffering and the passing of another human being, not least because it is a regular reminder that one day, it will be us for whom the bell is tolling.

The tolling referred to in Donne's quote is, of course, the ringing of funeral bells. The funeral bell that tolls for another person's death also tolls for us. Ernest Hemingway's masterwork about the Spanish Civil War was named *For Whom the Bell Tolls* after Donne's line, not just because death pervades the protagonist Robert Jordan's thoughts, but because the political and emotional reverberations of the war far transcended those of a national conflict, affecting the balance of nations.

Some authors clearly prefer to temper their "toll" by writing for specific audiences. For example, Brenda Bell Brown, one of the "multicultural writers" I referenced in the previous essay, is adamant about "writing Black" and in a manner that is firmly rooted in the Black American cultural tradition. Brown writes, "It is better for your sanity and your time to go into a project with a strong grasp of your intended audience and your commitment to their reading satisfaction. It saves you a lot of rewrite time even with all the technical aspects considered because, most importantly, it keeps the text true to you."

Brown is a woman of conviction who writes for a special purpose and audience and a standard of practice that does not apologize for being "too Black." Instead, her writing celebrates it! I prefer to write for a wider audience; yet, in line with Brown's philosophy, I keep my writing true to myself. Writers must decide for themselves how they want to position their narratives – for a narrowly tailored audience, or not. There is no right or wrong audience, no right or wrong essay "for whom the narrative tolls" as long as the writer holds true to their convictions, tells their story from their unique perspective, and uses their own true voice in communicating the story.

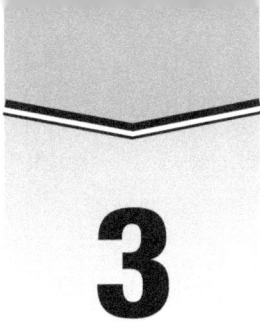

3

Opening Up

"Writing holds the potential for comfort and insight to come out of your difficult or painful experiences."
—John Fox

Here is what I know to be true: reading – close reading – and writing opens up a rewarding path for inquiry, reflection, understanding, and creativity that is ultimately healing.

The process of "opening up" is marvelous to watch, whether it's witnessed in psychotherapy or seen in nature. Flowers and plants, like people, come into bloom. New trees become part of the forest canopy. Even onions bloom!

Nature takes her time to "open up," and people do, too. People, like flowers, need time to emerge from their fragile bulbs and blossom. Once in bloom, they need to be nurtured.

Some people open up in tandem with nature: cyclical. After they open, they close for a period of time. They drop their petals and wither, only to blossom the following season. Perhaps they are perennials.

I've seen plants shut down due to insufficient nurturing, or a lack of rain or sunshine. Some plants are abused and neglected. Unlike perennials, whose regrowth is programmed, these plants do not open on cue. They are fragile. They need TLC.

Upon viewing wilted plants in my office, a patient said she could no longer see me. "If you can't take care of your plants," she sighed, "how do you expect to take care of me?"

Ultimately, nature, like people, are unpredictable. They are like large sections of forest that have been leveled by severe storms or landslides. Traumatic events in nature have the power to radically change the forest's appearance.

Traumatized people are no different. They may or may not be capable of regaining their footing, of repairing themselves, of returning to baseline. Like the forest, their character may be damaged forever.

I "opened up" late in life. You could say I was a "late bloomer." I walked and talked late. I entered puberty late. I was socially stunted and intellectually blunted.

I blossomed in medical school, graduating AΩA, and later, number one in my executive MBA program.

The point is that people open up at different times and under different circumstances. Children's brains mature at different rates, and some – not all – will become emotionally intelligent as well as natively intelligent.

Parents fret about their children and worry excessively, hoping one day they'll bloom – or maybe not ever, infantilizing them.

"Opening up" is a term I first encountered in psychotherapy, as a psychiatric resident. My analyst told me I was anxious because I put myself in my patients' shoes, a sign that I was "open" to their needs, perhaps even afraid of "catching" their hallucinations.

Medical students have similar fears, but not to that extreme. Students have exaggerated worries about their health. Maybe they, too, need therapy.

Whether you are in therapy, or are becoming a therapist, the process of "opening up" can be remarkable, if handled correctly. My analyst leaned forward, crossed his index fingers, and held them close to my face. "Art, you can empathize with your patients and I guarantee you will not catch their conditions."

What a gallant attempt to open me up – and it worked, for a while. Other fears set in that made it difficult for me to continue practicing. I closed down.

I think my analyst was correct: the entire process of "opening up" can resemble a psychedelic trip. The lines between reality, wish, and fantasy can easily become blurred. Strong emotions may even produce psychotic-like thoughts.

One of my supervisors said that the closest thing to psychosis that normal people experience is falling in love. He called it "the rush." The experience is very primordial, and it only lasts six months, he told us.

I have fallen in love. I have been in therapy. I have conducted therapy. I have lived to prove others wrong. Now I am learning to write from my heart.

All these efforts involve "opening up." None have caused me to "hear voices" or "see things." I am still grounded. My reality testing is good. I am loved by my family, and they love me.

My writing is less formal. I have freedom to be creative. I am comfortable using plain language. I write in a more conversational tone. I have embraced storytelling in my writing.

I have opened up.

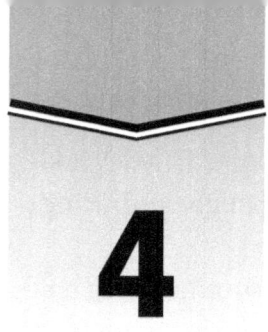

Why Aren't You Writing?

Don't wait for Halloween!

Sir Isaac Newton dedicated as much, if not more, of his time to the study of alchemy than he did to the natural order of the universe, but most of his work as an alchemist remained unpublished until long after his death when a metal chest full of his belongings was auctioned in 1936. The great man of science, the first of the Age of Reason, was simultaneously the last of the magicians.

To think that Newton may have thought more about levity than gravity seems absurd. It also explains why he couldn't or didn't publish much of his research; he would have needed a different physics and a different calculus to explain his findings. His peers would have thought him crazy, as if the apple that befell him did some brain damage.

Perhaps it is best that we keep some things to ourselves as personal secrets never to be shared, lest we are considered extremists, completely out of step with the times, or simply misunderstood. However, I suspect that the great majority of physicians have within them relevant literary contributions that they've been holding back, maybe written yet fearfully tucked away in a drawer.

Most physicians keep their thoughts and stories to themselves. Doctors feel they may be judged or criticized for their writing. Some believe they lack sufficient talent to be writers, while others insist they don't have the time to write. These are all excuses used by physicians who aspire to be narrative writers – excuses not to write. My advice to them is please do not let your great-great-great-grandchildren discover your unpublished ideas or manuscripts and sell them at auction. The time to write and publish is now. The question is: Why aren't you writing?

Writing is not rocket science. All of us have had to write narratives of some sort since grade school. Believe me, if I can do it, so can you. The reason I say this is because my fourth-grade writing assignment was to compose and illustrate a short fiction piece about Halloween. I remember writing about monsters and ghosts and clumsily outlining them and coloring them with crayons. I wanted the piece to be scary, so I chose a cemetery as the backdrop. The creatures were eyeing the candy of the trick-or-treaters in the cemetery – literally eying the candy. I drew them with big eyes, long before I became fascinated by psychiatry (schizophrenic patients will often draw eyes because they can constantly feel like they are being watched). My fatal flaw was not that the plot was ill-conceived – why should people be trick-or-treating in a cemetery? – or that my artistic ability was nil. Rather, in the story, I spelled the word "human being" incorrectly, writing "bean" instead of "being."

Now that word processing programs have spell check, spelling should not be a problem for anyone, although you still have to proofread your work because even in my example, "bean" may not have been detected as an improper spelling. Otherwise, the mechanics I aimed for in my fourth-grade story still apply: write to foster empathy and active listening and engage the audience in your narrative.

Here are some other basic principles you should consider when incorporating narrative medicine writing into your daily practice.

Pay attention to the patient's story, not just their symptoms. This includes their emotional state, their living conditions and lived experiences, their fears, and their hopes.

When taking patient histories, don't begin with, "What brings you here today?" Instead, ask, "What do you think I should know about your condition (or situation)?" Delve deeper than just the medical facts. Ask about their personal lives, their experiences with their illness, and how it affects their daily routines.

Keep a journal close by to write about your experiences and those of your patients or give yourself prompts and reminders to reflect upon later (see essay 6). Ponder patient interactions, your decisions, and your emotions. This can help you process your experiences and gain insights.

Read narratives and memoirs by other health care professionals (see essay 14). This can provide you with new perspectives and help you understand the value of narrative medicine. Practice close reading, i.e., looking at both what the text says (its content) and how the text says what it says – through imagery, figurative language, motif, and so on.

Consider participating in workshops or courses on narrative medicine. This can provide you with certain skills and knowledge to incorporate narrative medicine into your practice.

Encourage your team to share their experiences and reflections. This can foster empathy, improve communication, and promote a better understanding of patients.

Encourage your patients to share their stories. This can be in the form of verbal narratives, written stories, or even art and music (see essays 39 and 40). This can help you understand their experience better and provide more personalized care.

Narrative medicine is not just about storytelling. It's about using narratives to improve health care delivery and promote healing. It requires practice and patience, but the rewards can be significant.

One of the greatest compliments paid to me was by a prominent psychiatrist, and his remarks were about my writing. I had asked the psychiatrist to write the lead chapter for a book I was editing, and it was already under contract with a publisher. The psychiatrist was late in submitting his chapter, and on top of that, his manuscript was poorly written. I did a major revision of his chapter, staying true to his points but improving the flow, grammar, and syntax and inserting scientific references to bolster its credibility.

I mailed the new and improved manuscript to the psychiatrist for his approval. Several days later, he called me.

"Art," he said, "You're an alchemist."

"How do you mean," I asked.

"You know how to turn shit into gold!"

Newton may have been onto something after all.

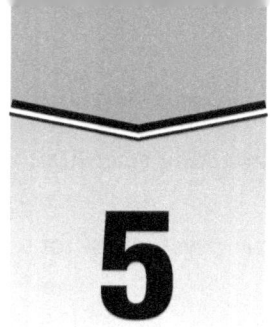

5

The Application of Creative Nonfiction to Medical Practice

When Oscar Wilde was asked how he spent his morning, he answered: *"I spent it revising a poem."*

"What changes did you make?"

"I took out a comma."

"What did you do in the afternoon?"

"I put it back."

Most writers have a preferred style of writing, using somewhat repetitive grammar, phrasing and syntax, choosing words that are familiar and seem reliable, ones that can be counted on to make their stories clear to readers. However, the best writing, in my opinion, shows the most variety; the writing is not predictable or redundant, and the writers are comfortable crossing genres. But just what are the main genres of narrative medicine writing?

First there is poetry. As I mentioned at the outset (essay 1), many of us have a jaundiced view of poetry based on antiquated notions and negative impressions, most gleaned from our formative years. Modern poetry today is quite different, however, and quite accessible. I could not do justice to its beauty in a short paragraph or two. Suffice it to say that poetry is the least rule-oriented form of writing. Detailed knowledge about poetic forms is fascinating and helpful, but it's not required for writing poetry. Ironically, that may explain why some doctors struggle writing poetry – it contradicts all the ways they were raised and trained: by rules, and with structure. The only rule in writing poetry – indeed, creative writing in general – is that there are no rules (or very few). What works, works. That's the science of it!

My narrative medicine instructor said that we change with every poem we write, and I do not think she was exaggerating. The Medici were fans of poetry and art for this reason. They saw it as a means to *renovatio* – to renew themselves and renovate humanity. My teacher then dispelled a myth. She said, "I know that so many conversations around poetry and writing are about 'revision.' Good writing is '10% inspiration and 90% perspiration.' It's not true!" Her advice to our class, and mine to you, is to write and just keep writing and you'll find that each new poem will reflect a new aspect of yourself. I recommend John Fox's *Poetic Medicine* as a good companion reader if you want to learn more about the "how to" of writing poetry.

At the opposite end of the writing spectrum is fiction. Physicians are natural storytellers by virtue of their training, recounting patients' detailed histories since medical school. The medical profession is rife with outstanding storytellers including W. Somerset Maugham, Sir Arthur Conan Doyle, Oliver Wendell Holmes, and Anton Chekhov, along with more contemporary authors such as Robin Cook, Michael Crichton, and Walker Percy.

Percy, a Columbia-trained physician best known for his philosophical novels set in and around New Orleans, remarked, "I was the happiest man ever to contract tuberculosis, because it enabled me to get out of Bellevue and quit medicine." Chekhov, a master of short stories, captured the appeal of writing fiction when he wrote: "Medicine is my lawful wife and literature my mistress; when I get tired of one, I spend the night with the other."

The fiction writer "Doug Zipes" – also Douglas P. Zipes, MD, Distinguished Professor Emeritus at Indiana University School of Medicine – is one of those physicians who has a mistress. He wrote: "I emphasized recently that life's journey is more important than the finish. This is particularly applicable to my late-blooming career in fiction ... Fiction allows for the creative freedom to invent your own universe, to imagine a world without boundaries, to conceive characters you love and make into heroes, or characters you hate that you can kill if you so choose. It is exhilarating and a world apart from writing tightly regulated science." Zipes has self-published four books of fiction and a memoir.

The sweet spot for me lies between poetry and fiction and is termed "creative nonfiction," which at first appears to be an oxymoron, but actually has deep literary roots. Lee Gutkind, author of *Keep It Real: Everything You Need to Know About Researching and Writing Creative Nonfiction*, is closely associated with this style of writing, "which presents or treats information using the tools of the fiction writer while maintaining allegiance to fact."

The creative nonfiction writing style tends to be dramatic and imaginative, but it never crosses the line into fiction because the content portrays a factually accurate account of real people and events, although in a compelling, vivid manner. "To put it another way," Gutkind explains, "creative nonfiction writers do not make things up; they make ideas and information that already exist more interesting and often more accessible ... Creative nonfiction writers have a complicated obligation to their readers: to entertain like novelists but to educate like journalists."

Narrative medicine writing is essentially creative nonfiction applied to medical practice. Narrative medicine employs techniques similar to creative nonfiction writing to tell stories and convey medical information. The application of creative nonfiction to medical practice can enhance the art of medicine and improve health outcomes. It can bridge the gap between science and humanity, and between physicians and patients. Creative nonfiction, like narrative medicine, can be applied in various other ways to enhance patient care, medical education, and research communication.

For example, creative nonfiction can be used to write patients' stories, which can help physicians better understand patients' experiences, perspectives, and emotions. This can lead to more empathetic care and improved patient satisfaction. It can also help patients better understand their own medical conditions and treatment plans. I wrote and published many case reports when I began my medical career. Although most of these reports leaned toward the rules of science and hence the writing style appeared rigid, creative liberties could be taken, for example, in describing the patient's personal, family and social history.

Creative nonfiction can be especially useful in medical education to teach students about the humanistic aspects of medicine. It can help students understand the psychological and social aspects of diseases and the impact of illnesses on patients' lives. This can lead to the development of more compassionate and holistic physicians. Writing programs have become wildly popular in medical schools, usually advertised under the banner of "narrative medicine," "creative writing," "reflective writing," and "creative nonfiction," attesting to the considerable overlap between these styles and categories.

Creative nonfiction can be used to communicate the results of medical research in a more accessible and engaging way. It can make complex medical information easier to understand and more relatable to a general audience. The best example is direct-to-consumer drug advertising, whether in print or on television. The results of clinical trials are presented to the audience in an impactful and memorable way, often with artistic and musical elements, yet the information conveyed must me accurate, truthful and not misleading.

For medical professionals, as I discussed in the previous essay, engaging in creative nonfiction/narrative medicine writing can serve as a form of reflection and self-care. It can help physicians process their experiences, cope with stress, and prevent burnout. A third of the students in my introductory class to narrative medicine were seasoned physicians. Some were on the verge of burnout or already there. But they eagerly looked forward to our weekly class sessions and were key participants.

Lastly, creative nonfiction can be used to convey public health messages in a more compelling way. It can help raise awareness about health issues and inspire people to take action. To give the public information on scientific issues that are complex and sometimes ethically contested, we must have writers who are skilled in presentation and have a thorough knowledge of medicine. Those who best fit that profile are doctors themselves.

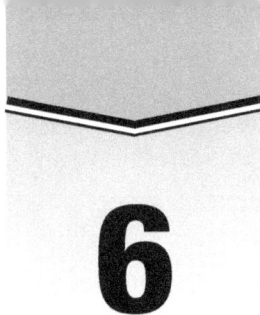

6

Reconstructing the Narrative

"Shine a ever lovin' light on me."
—John Fogerty (traditional, From "The Midnight Special"
   by Creedence Clearwater Revival)

I regret not keeping a diary or journal to write about patient encounters and interactions with peers, residents and attendings, not to mention the sundry characters connected to the academic health center where I trained and practiced. Had I done that, I would have had a lot more material to write about, and my depictions of events probably would have been more accurate.

With a world of rich clinical material in front of you, regardless where you practice, you will regret relying solely on your memory to write about patients and players you will meet along the way. The vignettes will seem fresher and will be more reliable when there is a permanent record of them, and your stories will be less affected by cognitive distortion wrought by time.

But even without the benefit of prompts or a written record, my career memories are very good, and my reconstruction of events is probably not affected by the vagaries of memory that can plague some writers (next essay).

I find myself gravitating toward short personal essays incorporating events that have special meaning to me and, I hope, to readers. I want these essays to have a moral or educational component to them, or at least a strong take-home message. My narratives could be considered memoir in that they often integrate material from an important time in my life. As I am typing this essay, for example, a memory from medical school erupts. Here is how the scene unfolds.

I am a fourth-year medical student on a family medicine elective in a community hospital located in a predominantly Black neighborhood. I am seriously dating a girl – she becomes my wife – and I am beginning to wear men's cologne. I am feeling good about life, making my mark (so I think), a survivor of my junior year of med school and cruising midway through my final year. I want people to notice me. I want to announce myself. I want to make a statement that I have "arrived." I want people to know I will soon be a doctor. I want to wear cologne.

It is lunch time in the clinic. My attending has disappeared. I am finishing my charting. The only other person is an elderly Black woman from housekeeping doing some light dusting. Earlier in the morning, I open the exam room door to examine a young Black male. I do not remember his chief complaint, but I do remember that when I take out my pen flashlight to see if his pupils are equal and reactive, he grabs the pen and flips it around, to shine a light on me. He also reaches for my stethoscope, which is dangling around my neck. He wants to examine me.

His affect is weird, and he brushes aside my questions. He isn't acting right. Putting it all together, I suspect he is in the midst of a psychotic episode. I excuse myself and inform my attending what is happening. He trusts my judgment – after all, I have completed two psych rotations, and my attending knows that I am going into psychiatry. The young man is sent to the emergency department to be further evaluated.

Why do I tell this story? Why does the memory suddenly occur in the fourth paragraph? I have told many stories about my medical training, but never this one. Perhaps the most important question is: is the story accurate?

In Patricia Hampl's book *I Could Tell You Stories*, one of her vignettes ("Memory and Imagination") describes a scene from early childhood in which her father drops her off at her first piano lesson. After providing intricate details of the scene, Hampl reflects, "No memoirist writes for long without experiencing an unsettling disbelief about the reliability of memory, a hunch that memory is not, after all, *just* memory." Upon reexamining her own account of the piano lesson, Hampl realizes that, although she tried to give a truthful version of the lesson, not all aspects of her story were accurate or even true. She would have written it differently if she had to do it over.

In narrative medicine, as with life, the truth of the events lies waiting in the details. I wonder how accurate are the details of my story, indeed all my stories? Was the stethoscope loose around my neck, or did I pull it from the pocket of my short white coat? Was it only the patients' affect that was bizarre, or did I do a full mental status examination and there were other abnormalities I have forgotten? Did my attending really trust my judgment (I would like to believe so), or did he do a cursory evaluation of the patient himself? I simply do not recall. And why, when I have retold some of my stories, have I repeated or written them slightly different than before? Why does it matter?

The answer is: the truth. As I stated in the previous essay, there are very few rules when it comes to writing medical narratives. But one rule that cannot be broken is that narrative medicine writing must be truthful. It may not always be accurate, but any inaccuracies cannot alter the truth. Lee Gutkind, author of *Keep it Real: Everything You Need to Know About Researching and Writing Creative Nonfiction*, stands firm on this point: "The writer cannot embellish, condense, or otherwise manipulate characters or events in order to make a more compelling story...The writer of creative nonfiction is bound, by an implicit and sometimes explicit contract with the reader, to make sure that the architecture of his story is based on authentic and reasonably verifiable experience."

Hampl writes, "I did not choose to remember the piano lesson. The experience was simply there." The same is true of my encounter with the patient: the memory merely trapsed forward, colored by my residual impression of it. But that's the risk of writing personal narratives without the benefit of transcription or source material: they are prone to inaccuracies. And that's why I wish I had kept a journal throughout my career – to rely less on my memory and more on a solid footing of events as they actually occurred.

According to Hampl, minor inventions to preserve the story do not necessarily make one a liar; rather, the need to reconstruct pieces of history forces us to admit that "memory is not a warehouse of finished stories, not a gallery of framed pictures." There is one thing I'll say, however, that I will always remember about that patient encounter, one undeniable, unshakable truth. The cleaning woman caught my gaze as I moved close to her. She smiled and said, "There's nothing I like better than a sweet-smelling man."

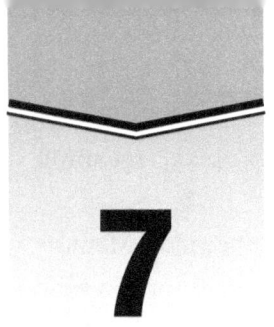

Incorporating Memoir in Narrative Medicine Writing

"Memoir is the intersection of narration and reflection, of storytelling and essay writing."
—Patricia Hampl

"This isn't a memoir, is it?" You're not asking me to publish your memoir, are you?" This was the reaction I received from an editor when pitching my previous collection of essays, *Every Story Counts*."

"Well, no, it definitely is not my memoir," I replied, "but yes, it does contain personal viewpoints and stories."

The word "memoir" originates from the French word "mémoire," which means "memory" or "reminiscence." The French term itself is derived from the Latin word "memoria," which also means "memory."

In English, the term "memoir" has been used since the 16th century to describe an individual's written account of their personal experiences and significant events in their life. It's a subset of the autobiographical genre, but it differs from an autobiography in that it usually focuses on a specific period or events in the author's life, rather than their entire life chronologically.

I think the harsh reaction I received from the editor was based on her thinking that memoir and autobiography are the same – they're clearly not. I was proposing a book of essays, some containing memoir.

(The word "essay" comes from the French word "essai," meaning "trial" or "attempt.")

Memoirs and personal essay collections are quite popular. Memoir writing – despite what William Grimes said in a critique for the *New York Times* (March 25, 2005), "We All Have a Life. Must We All Write About It?" – is not necessarily a bad thing. There are many wonderful, human, funny, and true stories out there. Individual stories, told well, have the power to change the world.

In *Keep It Real*, Lee Gutkind observes: "Memoir writing is not about self-obsession, even though the subject is invariably the experience of one life. Good memoirs should do what all good art aspires to do. They show us ourselves. This is arguably the distinction between good and bad memoir writing. Bad memoirs often offer readers the book equivalent of reality TV."

I wasn't asking the editor to publish my life's version of "Love After Lockup" or "The Real Housewives of..." And I certainly was not suggesting anything as salacious as "Naked and Afraid." The point is that bad memoir writing, like bad television, is self-indulgent and involves excessive contemplation of oneself or a single issue at the expense of a wider view and audience.

Gutkind continues, "A good memoir offers readers a human connection. A good memoir writer uses life experience, not to go more deeply into the self but to reach out to others. A good memoirist makes connections. A good memoirist's primary goal is to show us something true about ourselves, about what it means to be human ... Individual human experience is valuable – in writing and elsewhere – only when it moves through, then transcends the self and connects to what's human in us all."

Gutkind's message is what was on my mind when I pitched my book to the editor. Fortunately, a different editor was on my wavelength, although she also balked until I sent her a dozen essays and an outline of the book. I understood her hesitancy, not only because there are bad memoirs, but also because incorporating memoir in narrative medicine writing can have several disadvantages. First, however, I'll mention the advantages:

Pros:

1. **Personal Perspective**: Because memoirs provide a personal viewpoint, they allow physicians to share their unique experiences and insights. It can help them reflect on their practice, decisions, and interactions with patients.
2. **Improved Empathy**: Writing memoirs can enhance a physician's empathy as they delve deeper into their feelings and reactions. It can help them understand their patients' experiences better.
3. **Healing Process**: It can be therapeutic for physicians as they process their experiences, particularly those involving trauma, loss, or ethical dilemmas, through writing.
4. **Education and Training**: Memoirs can serve as valuable resources for teaching and training in medical schools, providing real-life examples and insights.
5. **Connection with Others**: Sharing memoirs can help connect physicians with their colleagues, fostering a sense of community and shared experiences.

Cons:

1. **Privacy Concerns**: Writing memoirs might involve sharing intimate details about patients, potentially breaching their privacy. Even when anonymized, there could be ethical implications.
2. **Subjectivity**: Memoirs, by nature, are subjective and may not present an objective or comprehensive view of medical events or practices.

3. **Time-Consuming**: Depending on the length, writing memoirs can be time-consuming, which might be challenging for busy physicians.

4. **Emotional Distress**: Delving into personal experiences, especially those that are traumatic or stressful, can cause emotional distress and trigger flashbacks and unpleasant details of clinical events.

5. **Potential Misinterpretation**: Readers might misinterpret the memoirs, leading to misunderstandings or misconceptions about the medical profession or specific practices.

Physician writers of medical memoir can be just as guilty of self-absorption as other kinds of writers of memoir, but medical memoir can also be an important tool for forging connections and healing bonds among doctors and patients. Physician memoirs offer inspiring accounts of life in medicine and medicine in life.

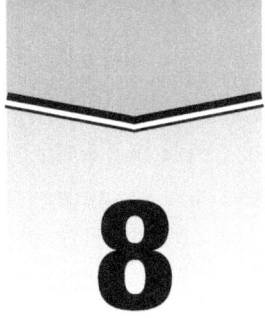

8

Exploring the Connection Between Creativity and Narrative Medicine Writing

Dear Vincent,

I hope this message finds you in good health despite your recent self-inflicted injury. The purpose of this letter is to discuss the intriguing relationship between creativity and narrative medicine writing. You told me you were certain such a link existed because you have witnessed a similar relationship among painters like yourself.

Let me digress a moment for the sake of our readers.

Narrative medicine writing is a form of writing that tells a factual story – usually about a patient – creatively, in a structured manner. Presumably there is a significant link between creativity and narrative medicine writing as there is in the realm of literature in general. Creativity fuels narrative writing by providing unique ideas and perspectives. It allows the writer to think outside of the box and to create a compelling, engaging narrative that captures the reader's attention.

Creativity can manifest in medical narratives in various forms. For instance, it can bring a complex, multi-dimensional patient to life or describe unexpected events in the patient's history inventively and artistically. It can also be reflected in the way the writer uses language to convey emotions, set the scene, or describe physicians, caregivers and family members central to the narrative.

Moreover, creativity in narrative medicine writing can enhance the reader's experience by making the narrative more vivid and engaging. It can lead to a deeper understanding and appreciation of the narrative by providing new insights and perspectives.

So, Vincent, now you know that creativity does, in fact, play a crucial role in narrative medicine writing, just as it does in painting and countless other mediums of self-expression. Creativity fuels engaging, thought-provoking narratives and enhances the reader's experience. Hence, nurturing creativity is essential for anyone involved in narrative writing.

How does one nurture creativity, you ask? You're under the impression that creativity is a trait we are born with – either we have it or we don't? And isn't there a connection between creativity and mental illness? You deem yourself expert on this topic, do you not, Vincent?

I can't give you definitive answers to all of those questions. Scholars have researched and written books about creativity, yet many points of contention remain. What I can say is that creativity can be practiced and learned to a degree. Everyone's creative process is unique, and each of us employs a combination of elements – some learned and others probably innate – to express what we want to write. Narrative writers also have tools that they learn how to apply to express their thoughts on paper.

For many writers – myself included – the element of surprise sparks creativity. Surprise rolls in like a tidal wave, totally unpredictable, when, like you, I am filling in my canvass yet not really knowing what should come next. Suddenly I surprise myself with a thought or a memory that, like a spark, catches fire and leads to something novel and creative. This moment of surprising myself as I write – or as you paint, I suspect – provides guidance: it reminds us where we have been and leads us to where we are going.

For example – and please forgive me Vincent for making this confession – I didn't originally intend to write to you. I began this letter with "Dear Reader" instead of "Dear Vincent," intending it for a general audience. I changed the salutation when I suddenly thought of you as I paused to reflect on creativity as it applies not only to writers but also to artists. How could I not think of you at such a time given that your mind is the embodiment of creativity, albeit driven toward unpredictable and self-destructive impulses.

I've read many accounts about your maladies, Vincent, and your doctors have given you a host of psychiatric diagnoses, most of them tainted by your excessive consumption of absinthe. Whatever mental affliction you may suffer, your moodiness seems to contribute to both your brilliance and baffling disorganization, which is evident in your paintings.

Perhaps you will find comfort in knowing that researchers have found connections between mood disorders – specifically bipolar disorder – and creativity: bipolar traits have been associated with enhanced creative expression in various occupations. Conversely, creativity plays a role in psychiatric treatment. Studies have shown that music and art therapy can be helpful for patients with schizophrenia, depression, and other mental disorders.

In summary, Vincent, I will say that narrative medicine writers tap into their creativity to reflect on their experiences as healers and the healed. They recognize that creativity is the process that blends medicine with the art and humanities. Their output is, ultimately, a story that can be shared with communities they care for. The question as to whether a connection exists between creativity and narrative medicine writing is perhaps best examined further by delving into its corollary: is storytelling hard-wired into our brains?

I'll follow up on that line of thinking in the next essay. That's all for now.

With warm regards,
Art Lazarus

P.S. Two of my singer-songwriter friends, Michael Franks and Don McLean, send their regards. Michael expresses empathy for your recent struggles. He has composed two songs for you: "Vincent's Ear" and "The Yellow House." In the former, Michael says no one understands all the love inside you tried to give, how hard your life was to live – a past which you could not desert – and a heart that was hurt somehow by someone. Michael regrets that your brief time with Paul Gauguin in the yellow house in Arles was a disaster, although you painted sunflowers, and your relationship to Paul was akin to a brother. Regrettably, Michael says it was "not enough to distract you from the end." Likewise, Don wants you to know:

> *"You took your life, as lovers often do*
> *But I could've told you, Vincent*
> *This world was never meant for*
> *One as beautiful as you"*

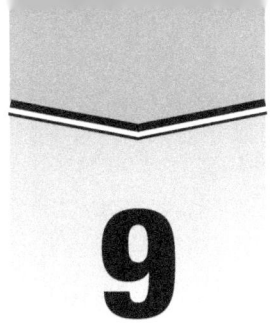

9

Is Storytelling Hard-Wired into Our Brains?

"Hey, did you hear the one about…?"
"How about a good bedtime story…?"
"You're not gonna believe this, but…"
"Can you tell me…"

Why, throughout human history, have people been so drawn to stories? Could it be because stories are first and foremost a survival mechanism? From an evolutionary standpoint, storytelling was a way to pass down vital information to ensure survival. Our ancestors shared stories to warn each other about dangers, share successful hunting strategies, or explain the world around them. This instinct to share and receive information through stories still drives our behavior – and it is indeed hard-wired into our brains.

In *The Sacred Balance: Rediscovering Our Place in Nature*, David Suzuki notes that our knack for narrative enables our ancestors to recognize, understand, and remember the meaning of patterns in nature, such as the migration of animals, the sequencing of the seasons, and the duration of night and day. In essence, the mind is telling itself a story aided by neural pathways constantly rewiring themselves to order sensory input.

Our stories, when jotted down on paper, become narratives. Our brains are programmed to learn and understand better through narratives. Telling stories and reading narratives activates many parts of the brains, sometimes for days. Whether you want your narrative to motivate, persuade or simply entertain, start with a story of human struggle – which is perfect for health narratives – and end it triumphantly. It will capture your readers hearts – by first attracting their brains.

Stories provide a structure that our minds easily comprehend and remember. They allow us to make sense of complex information by placing it in a context we can understand. One estimate suggests that we can recall facts up to 22 times more effectively when they are part of a story rather than just isolated data. So, if you want a fact to stick, the best thing to do is explain it with a story.

"The Epic of Gilgamesh" is perhaps the oldest written story on earth – a poem, actually, of adventure-filled tales. It is based on the real historical King of Uruk, Gilgamesh, who reigned around 2700 BC. The text we know today was written approximately 2100 BC and discovered on 12 clay tablets in cuneiform script in the mid-19th century. The fragments of the tablets were unearthed by archeologists in excavations across what is now Syria and Iraq, and they were painstakingly restored. The young man who decoded the tablets' puzzle was an English archaeologist named George Smith working for the British Museum.

Despite the date and place of its origin, the exploits of Gilgamesh showcase many of the same elements and themes still present in the stories enjoyed today by modern readers – a hero embarks on a difficult journey in which there is romance and seduction, encounters with strange and exotic characters, and impossible obstacles to overcome. Along the way, Gilgamesh rubs elbows with the gods and searches for the key to immortality – all with predictably tragic results. In a refrain that remains true today, the narrator remarks that no one truly dies as long as they are remembered by the living.

It is not a coincidence that the epic's themes of friendship, the fear of death, the pursuit of knowledge, and the search for immortality bear similarities to contemporary stories. Time does not seem to matter much to themes; nor indeed does location. A 2006 analysis of 90 folktale collections from around the world (from both tribal societies and industrialized ones) reveals as much, with scholars describing the presence of a number of distinctly common narratives covering basic human needs and desires in the stories they examined.

In *The Seven Basic Plots: Why We Tell Stories*, the late journalist and author Christopher Booker reasoned there are just seven of these universal plots, and they can be seen time and again in books, television shows, movies and even podcasts. They are:

1. **Overcoming the Monster** - *The War of the Worlds, Star Wars, Jaws*
2. **Rags to Riches** - *Cinderella, Jane Eyre, The Prince and the Pauper*
3. **The Quest** - *The Iliad, The Lord of the Rings, Raiders of the Lost Ark*
4. **Voyage and Return** – *Alice's Adventures in Wonderland, The Time Machine, Gulliver's Travels*
5. **Comedy** - *A Midsummer Night's Dream, Four Weddings and a Funeral, The Big Lebowski*
6. **Tragedy** - *Hamlet, The Great Gatsby, Citizen Kane*
7. **Rebirth** – *Groundhog Day, A Christmas Carol, The Shawshank Redemption*

Almost all stories can be simplified into one of these core themes. All categories engage our primal emotions and trigger and stimulate the release of neurochemicals like cortisol, dopamine, endorphins, and especially oxytocin, referred to as the "bonding hormone" or "love hormone." Compelling narratives cause oxytocin release and have the power to affect our attitudes, beliefs and behaviors. Oxytocin is also released in high amounts during childbirth and is believed to enhance empathy and emotional connections. This emotional engagement makes stories more memorable and impactful.

Simply telling stories can increase our empathy towards others we may have initially viewed as outsiders. That's why stories are a fundamental part of our social interactions and why storytelling has been an important tool for social cohesion for millennia: they allow us to share our experiences, understand others' perspectives, and foster connections. It's no surprise that social gatherings often revolve around the sharing of stories. In fact, it's estimated that as much as 65% of all human interactions take the form of social storytelling (i.e., gossip).

Stories stimulate our imagination and creativity. They allow us to explore different scenarios, solve problems, and think creatively, all of which are necessary for narrative writers. With around a hundred billion neurons and almost a quadrillion connections between the neurons in our brains, the organ borders on the wondrous, just like our stories. Yet, for all its complexity, the brain is still a pattern-seeking instrument that looks to put the chaos of the world into some kind of recognizable order.

Perhaps that is what the beloved Sufi scholar and poet Jalaluddin Rūmī understood when he wrote, "What you seek is seeking you."

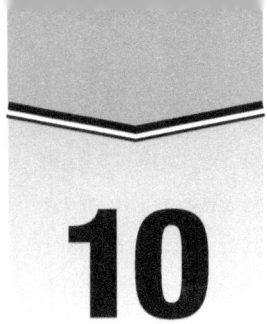

10

Was Munchausen the Ultimate Storyteller?

"The lies that people tell in stories is what makes them so true."
— Majid Kazmi

"The Epic of Gilgamesh" may be one of the earliest works of literature in the world, but surely the greatest storyteller of all time was Baron Hieronymus Karl Friedrich von Münchhausen (1720-1797), a German calvary officer.

The stories told by Baron Munchausen were fantastic and absurd, often featuring impossible achievements. They are a classic example of tall tales and the tradition of hyperbolic storytelling. Here are a few examples:

1. On a hunting trip, the Baron claims to have ridden on a cannonball, flown to the moon, and been swallowed by a giant fish, from which he escaped by tickling it with a feather.
2. In another tale, he pulls himself (and his horse) out of a swamp by his own hair.
3. In yet another story, he tells of a time when he was traveling in winter, and his horse was frozen in place overnight. When it was cut free, the horse was accidentally severed in half, and the half with the head and front legs ran off, only to return in spring perfectly healthy and whole.

The tales of Baron Munchausen have become a part of popular culture, referenced in a variety of media and spawning the term "Munchausen" to characterize pathological liars. Munchausen syndrome is familiar to doctors because it describes a psychiatric disorder in which someone pretends to be ill or deliberately produces symptoms of illness in themselves or others ("Munchausen by proxy"). Munchausen patients are bent on deceiving physicians by their conscious production of signs and symptoms of physical illness – and for no apparent gain other than to assume the patient role.

One of the characteristic features of Munchausen's syndrome is a tendency for patients to give a false but plausible history and seek out caregivers by wandering from hospital to hospital. They often demand hospitalization and request invasive diagnostic procedures and sometimes surgery. Although these patients are generally not suicidal or have a death wish, a few have died in surgery.

I was consulted on several cases of patients suspected of having Munchausen's syndrome. I say "suspected" because the syndrome is nearly impossible to prove unless patients are caught in the act of fabricating their illness – for example, by pricking their finger and squeezing a few drops of blood into their urine specimen to simulate hematuria. When confronted with their surreptitious behavior, Munchausen patients typically deny it and move on, signing out of the hospital against medical advice.

Munchausen's syndrome was so-named by the British endocrinologist Richard Asher in 1951. Asher observed: "Like the famous Baron von Munchausen, the persons affected have always traveled widely; and their stories, like those attributed to him, are both dramatic and untruthful." The term "Munchausen's syndrome" is probably a misnomer, however, since the Baron himself was never chronically ill nor did he feign illness.

Asher considered Munchausen's syndrome to be similar to the Walter Mitty syndrome, in reference to the popular short story, "The Secret Life of Walter Mitty," in which the protagonist is engaged in never-ending reverie. James Thurber, creator of the Walter Mitty character (famously played on screen originally by Danny Kaye and later by Ben Stiller), commented: "The original of Walter Mitty is every other man I have ever known. When the story was printed in the *New Yorker* [March 18, 1939] six men from around the country, including a Des Moines dentist, wrote and asked me how I had got to know them so well. No writer can ever put his finger on the exact inspiration of any character in fiction that is worthwhile, in my estimation. Even those commonly supposed to be taken from real characters rarely show much similarity in the end."

Unraveling the Munchausen legend has proven as challenging as the patients themselves. Apparently, the author of the Munchausen stories was not Munchausen himself but instead Rudolf Erich Raspe (1737-1794), also of dubious character. Accused of embezzlement, Raspe fled Europe disguised as a Dutchman and settled in London. Raspe anonymously published *Baron Munchausen's Narrative of His Marvelous Travels and Campaigns in Russia* in 1785. The book initially sold poorly, but after another publisher assumed responsibility for the printing, many volumes followed in rapid succession, all expanding on the original version.

Raspe's biographer, John Carswell, believed the Munchausen stories were actually an exaggeration of Raspe's own life, a projection of his "frustrated egotism." Raspe probably knew Munchausen, however, since they were both from the same area of Germany. Munchausen died three years after Raspe, a humiliated and bitter man despite achieving celebrity status. Munchausen never discovered the identity of the man who brought him unwelcome fame, that is, Raspe, whose antisocial behavior and fugitive existence was a facsimile of the typical Munchausen patient.

This tale is for real!

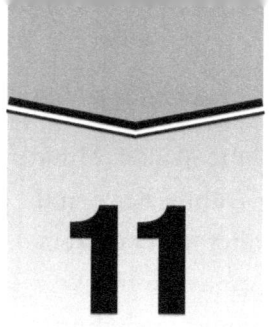

11

The Empowering Hermann Hesse

Find the way to yourself.

I am not a philosopher, and I do not pretend to know the meaning of life or whether humas are destined to have a purpose or higher order other than procreation. But I've frequently thought about this philosophical issue.

I first questioned the meaning of life when I was in high school. Mind you, I was a typical teenager interested in sports and the opposite sex, and I was not a particularly deep thinker. All that changed when I read two books by Hermann Hesse: *Beneath the Wheel* and *Demian*. The latter included a passage that forever changed my outlook on life and gave me a true sense of purpose at a time when I really was not searching for one.

In Hesse's coming of age novel, *Demian*, the protagonist, Emil Sinclair, has an epiphany. He exclaims, "I wanted only to live in accord with the promptings which came from my true self. Why was that so very difficult?" This quote is frequently cited by readers as having very deep meaning for them. Indeed, here I am, recently turned 70, and I'm still asking myself why those true promptings are still so tricky to navigate.

There was a passage in *Demian* – a passage where Sinclair reflects on his growth and discovering himself – that left quite an impression on me, and this passage became a guiding theme throughout my life:

> "I did not exist to write poems, to preach or to paint, neither I nor anyone else. All of that was incidental. Each man had only one genuine vocation – to find the way to himself. He might end up as a poet or madman, as a prophet or criminal – that was not his affair, ultimately it was of no concern. His task was to discover his own destiny – not an arbitrary one – and live it out wholly and resolutely within himself. Everything else was only a would-be existence, an attempt at evasion a flight back to the ideals of the masses, conformity and fear of one's own inwardness. [...]
>
> I was an experiment on the part of Nature a gamble within the unknown, perhaps for a new purpose, perhaps for nothing, and my only task was to allow this game on the part of primeval depths to take its course, to feel its will within me and make it wholly mine. That or nothing!"

Upon graduating medical school, I was literally given a blank canvass in my yearbook to do anything I wanted with "my page" – write something, thank people, show photographs of family and friends, etc. I chose to include thank-yous and photographs like most of my classmates, but I also included that passage from *Demian*. It was my motto, my creed, my way of remembering that I could end up a "madman" by entering the field of psychiatry – and I nearly did!

Now, ironically, nearing the end of my life (statistically, that is), I find myself becoming transfixed on prose and poetry. Writing seems to have become *my* genuine vocation. And I do not think Hesse would have objected. Although he is best known for his novels, Hesse was also a poet. In the seven volume German edition of his works, there are approximately 480 pages of poems. Hesse's novels themselves contain many passages of literal verse. Here is what Hesse said about poets and poems:

"In its origin a poem is something completely unequivocal. It is a discharge, a call, a cry, a sigh, a gesture, a reaction by which the living soul seeks to defend itself from or to become aware of an emotion, an experience. In this first spontaneous, most important function no poem can be judged. It speaks first of all simply to the poet himself, it his cry, his scream, his dream, his smile, his whirling fists."

Hesse was a prophetic voice of the 20th century. He captivated readers with his philosophical and introspective writing. His great works reflected his own experiences in life along with an accounting of human values and morals. By exploring the way people are affected by their station in life, Hesse was a master at dissecting themes of self-discovery, spirituality, and the pursuit of authenticity. His novels are timeless. In fact, *Demian* was originally published (in 1919) under the pseudonym "Emil Sinclair," and it was subtitled *The Story of a Youth*, to give the impression that "youth" could be a single person or a generation – any generation.

What endears me the most to Hesse, however, is his universal acceptance of people for who they are and what they do, in recognition of their equality and the uniqueness of each individual person. His writing is non-judgmental, allowing creativity to flow unfettered, and appreciating the essence of life as it is. Hesse claims (in *My Beliefs*) that "no poem can be bad enough," observing: "The reading of bad poems is always a short-term pleasure; you quickly get enough of it. So why read? Cannot anyone make bad poems for himself? Try it sometime and you will find that making bad poems actually gives much more pleasure than reading even the most beautiful ones."

How encouraging and empowering that Hesse would not condemn bad poetry and simply say write it yourself.

That's what I do. I write bad poems!

12

Man's Search for Meaning is Spiritual, and Relevant to Medicine

Frankl's Holocaust memoir should be on everyone's must-read list.

Viktor Frankl's psychological study of the Holocaust, *Man's Search for Meaning*, is an extraordinary essay on resilience and spirituality, a reminder that human life, under any circumstances, never ceases to have meaning. At the risk of mentioning Bob Dylan in the same sentence as Viktor Frankl, it was Dylan who said: "When you ain't got nothing, you got nothing to lose." I suppose Bob Dylan read the book too, ranked by the Library of Congress as "one of the ten most influential books in America.

Man's Search for Meaning is as much about hope as it is about loss. "Whoever was still alive had reason for hope," Frankl told his comrades. They could hope for health, family, happiness, fortune, and a return to their occupation and position in society. "After all, we still had our bones intact," Frankl reasoned. Clearly, he set the bar low.

Anyone searching for a meaning to their life will be disappointed if they think they will have it after reading Frankl's book. Frankl specifically writes that the meaning of life cannot be defined in a general way, because it "differ[s] from man to man, and from moment to moment." Nor can the meaning of life be answered by "sweeping statements." A person's unique opportunity – the reason for their existence – lies in the way in which they bear their burden. Indeed, the words over the entrance gate to Auschwitz concentration camp – Arbeit Macht Frei – meant: "Work Sets You Free." Even under the most difficult circumstances such as forced labor, Frankl would have seen a deeper meaning to it.

In contrast to Emil Sinclair's epiphany uncovered in *Demian* in the previous essay, i.e., the realization that: "Each man had only one genuine vocation – to find the way to himself" – Frankl was of the persuasion that "it did not matter what we expected from life, but rather what life expected of us." Individuals content with the life they lead and forgiving of their own flaws may not be able to learn much from *Man's Search for Meaning*, for Frankl would have us believe that it is important to overcome adversity and hardship to derive meaning in life. Frankl speaks not only of hard labor and the day-to-day unknowing of whether one would be executed or gassed, but also the ability to withstand the brutal pain of disease and famine. Common among the prisoners were malnutrition (~200 calories/day), severe vitamin deficiencies, lice infestations, frostbite and typhus outbreaks.

Epidemic typhus is caused by a bacterium (Rickettsia prowazekii) spread to people through contact with infected body lice. Though epidemic typhus was responsible for millions of deaths in previous centuries, it is now considered a rare disease. Occasionally, cases continue to occur, in areas where extreme overcrowding is common and body lice can travel from one person to another.

The concentration camps were a different story; they were fertile ground for the spread of typhus. The exact number of prisoners who contracted typhus cannot be determined, but the number has been estimated at well over 100,000. Frankl became infected with typhus and almost died. The first symptoms, visible several days after infection, were high fever and a rash. Next came damage to the central nervous and circulatory systems, including delirium and myocarditis.

Effective treatment with antibiotics was not available during World War II, and a lack of nutrition made it harder for a prisoner's immune system to fight off disease. Mass selection of infected prisoners for the gas chambers was a common method of "prevention." Recovery without treatment occurred after about four weeks for the lucky few, although to be sure, many did not consider themselves lucky to survive the ordeal, believing they would be better off dead.

One has to wonder how those who were not killed upon arrival at the camps managed to survive. They were condemned to unimaginable torment – both physical and psychological – as well as to a sense of constant insecurity about their future, starvation, labor beyond their capacity, and utterly unsanitary living conditions that fostered the spread of numerous infectious diseases (not only typhus). On this point, Frankl quotes Nietzsche – "He who has a *why* to live for can bear with any *how*" – and concludes that "only the men who allowed their hold on their moral and spiritual selves to subside eventually fell victim to the camp's degenerating influences." However, not many were capable of reaching great spiritual heights, which Frankl conceded was man's meaning in life even if spirituality was experienced differently by each person.

There is a parallel between Frankl's world and the medical world, where patients have survived grave medical illnesses associated with grim prognoses. Research has shown that spirituality often provides a coping mechanism for individuals facing severe illnesses. Conversely, a decline in spirituality seems to be associated with potentially negative health effects.

For example, a spiritual life can offer comfort, improve resilience, and provide a sense of purpose, which may enhance the overall quality of life and even positively influence survival rates. Spirituality can influence health behaviors like adherence to medication, diet, and exercise regimens, which can significantly affect the outcomes of patients with grave illnesses.

Patients who engage in spiritual practices may experience less anxiety, depression, and stress, which can positively affect their overall health status and potentially their prognosis. Some studies suggest a potential link between spirituality and the immune system. Patients with strong spiritual beliefs may experience less inflammation and improved immune response, which could potentially impact their ability to combat serious illnesses.

As a physician and psychiatrist, Frankl was keenly aware of the impact of the prisoners' physical and mental states on their survival: they were highly correlated. In other words, prisoners who were better able to withstand the mental and physical torture were more likely to survive partly due to a healthier immune system and fewer depressive and suicidal thoughts. In this context, it is worth noting that spirituality can also play a crucial role in end-of-life care, influencing decisions about treatments and interventions. It can lead to better patient satisfaction and potentially improved survival rates.

It is also important to note that while these correlations exist, the relationship between spirituality and health is complex and influenced by a variety of factors. More research is needed to fully understand the mechanisms behind these associations.

NARRATIVE IN EDUCATION, TRAINING & PRACTICE

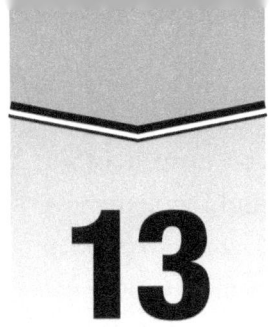

13

Enhancing Practice Through the Narrative

Writing benefits medical students and busy practitioners alike.

When I enrolled in a narrative medicine program at a local university, my first homework assignment was to "write 800 words." No topic was specified. I had the freedom to write about anything that could reasonably be construed as narrative medicine writing, which, according to Rita Charon, MD, PhD a general internist who is synonymous with the narrative medicine movement, is medicine that incorporates writing with the clinical skills of recognizing, absorbing, interpreting, and being moved by the stories of patients' illnesses.

Charon, who is the executive director of the narrative medicine program at Columbia University, considers narrative medicine a basic science mandatory for medical practice. Narrative-based practice works in two ways. First, it uses literary texts and storytelling to improve the empathic ability of students, teaching them to become better listeners. Second, by incorporating a narrative pedagogy into the medical school curriculum and helping students process their clinical experiences through writing assignments, narrative medicine fortifies clinical practice.

Excluding my two-year stint in an executive MBA program in the mid-1990s, I haven't had a homework assignment since I graduated college nearly 50 years ago. I never considered reading assignments in medical school as "homework." Medical school never offered me the option of picking and choosing a topic to study or, heaven forbid, figuring out ways to make education less stressful and fun somehow. Perhaps that is why narrative medicine writing has become so popular among medical students: It restores value to the subjective experience of suffering that is often lost in the objective way students are taught and trained.

Narrative medicine is now taught in some form at approximately 80% of medical schools in the United States: courses, seminars, workshops and graduate degree programs. Programs are designed for students and seasoned practitioners alike. Some are led by physicians, some by journalists, and many by individuals with advanced degrees in creative writing. Practically all programs have in common mechanisms to improve clinical care through narratives.

Narrative medicine classes for medical students are not meant to replace lecture-based classes but instead supplement them, e.g., through elective courses or didactics interwoven longitudinally with traditional courses and clerkships. Narrative medicine programs have reported numerous benefits, including decreasing burnout in students. Narrative medicine claims to increase students' confidence and instill a strong patient-centered focus. Early exposure to the principles and practice of narrative medicine – as early as the first semester of medical school – may enhance professional development by fostering self-awareness, competency building, mindfulness, and spiritualism and humanism. Research on this burgeoning field is ongoing.

The importance of writing narratives and the benefits that accrue to medical students in particular cannot be understated in light of the empathy and compassion fatigue that begin to set in halfway through medical school, precisely when students embark on their clinical rotations and emotional responsiveness is required to assist patients through difficult times. However, after two intense years of rigorous scientific studies replete with courses that sap the life out of most medical students, it's not easy to set them free in clinical settings and tell them to "be themselves" and "be attentive" to patients. Many students are already burned out, depressed – even suicidal – and feel like imposters. But that's the hidden beauty of the narrative: reflection and writing not only helps students connect to their patients, it allows them to connect to themselves, fostering self-expression in genuine ways. Like ice caps melting, new identities emerge, long submerged under the weight of textbooks and the influence of med-speak. Writing can counter the trauma of the initial and subsequent years of medical education and training.

Medical students are not judged when they write – or at least they should not be judged. They are not critiqued, put down or pimped by attendings in authority. Students are allowed to take risks, and they can make mistakes in narrative healthcare programs. Medical practice, on the other hand, is unforgiving; it requires constant perfection. Any deviation from practice guidelines requires a thorough explanation, and even then, a novice engaging in the "art" of medicine – practice based on individual experience rather than peer-reviewed guidelines – is likely to be frowned upon. Practicing medicine tests your nerves and readily shakes your confidence; writing builds self-esteem and strengthens confidence.

My hope is that medical students, residents and physicians will consider taking a course or two in narrative medicine. Given the virtually infinite number of options and arrangements to choose from, courses will accommodate the schedules and preferences of most applicants, ranging from medical students to busy practitioners. The program that interested me the most offered a "certificate" after completing three graduate-level courses. Each course occurred via distance learning – two hours, online – the same evening each week for a semester. If, for any reason, students missed a class, they could view a video of it at their leisure before the next class. The courses that appealed to me were roughly divided into the following topics:

- Writing assignments and engagement with narrative prose and poems.

- Studies of illness narratives in poetry, short fiction, creative nonfiction, and novels.
- Studies of narratives by doctors and other healthcare providers, with an emphasis on reflective writing skills.

The value of narrative medicine should be obvious: courses extend naturally to clinical practice and help physicians become better attuned to the contexts of their patients' needs and distress. Integrating narratives into clinical practice also helps optimize physicians' well-being and restore meaning in work.

14

Achieving Literary Competence in Medical Students

Start reading. The choices are endless.

During my college years, I took two English courses: English composition (required), and world literature related to mental illness: a course aptly titled "Madness and Folly as Mirrors of Man Before the Age of Reason." With only these two courses, I was ahead of most of my medical school classmates in literary competence. It's a sad commentary on the weight given to the role of literature in preparation for medical school and a life thereafter.

Achieving literary competency in medical students aims to understand, appreciate, and use literature to enhance their professional development and improve patient care. It involves understanding that literature can provide valuable insights into the human experience of illness, health, and healthcare. Literature can provide medical students with a broader perspective on the human condition and the doctor-patient relationship.

In a classic study published in *Academic Medicine* in 1989, "Unmet Needs and Unused Skills: Physicians' Reflections on their Liberal Arts Education," physicians who graduated from three top-notch small liberal arts colleges between 1955 and 1982 were surveyed and said they wished they had taken more courses in the humanities – not only English literature, but also art, history and music – to better prepare them for dealing with practice and the vicissitudes of patient care. The greatest unmet need was reported to be "skill with people."

One of the conclusions reached by the study authors was that "the daily practice of medicine, in most cases, does not require immense scientific sophistication." Yet medical schools have scoffed at the idea of teaching humanities due to the constant growth of scientific and new medical advancements. Fortunately, progressive medical school admission committees now select more well-rounded college students, including applicants who have been exposed to literature and the humanities. Admission committees claim that exposure to literature can help develop a critical eye and research skills, as well as introduce students to ideas, cultures and views they may otherwise miss. Still, there are those who assert that the study of literature has goals and purposes unrelated to the medical profession, and that a strong science background should prevail.

I beg to disagree. Medical students need to be competent not only in the natural sciences but also in the social sciences and the humanities in order to converse intelligently with a heterogeneous health-conscious public. Literacy study can enrich medical students' moral education, foster a tolerance for the uncertainties of clinical practice, and provide a grounding for empathic attention to patients. Stories, essays, first-person narratives, and poetry also facilitate the professional identity formation of medical students. Ultimately, the development of medical professionalism will benefit from the critical and interrogative methods of literature.

It is not impossible for medical students to undertake a premedical curriculum that offers both scientific and literary competencies. The time to start reading, however, is in high school, continuing (or catching up) in college, and devoting additional time to close reading in medical school, residency and practice. Unless scholarly works from the humanities – including literature among other disciplines – become part of the educational repertoire of physicians, they will fail to achieve the ideals embraced in the practice of medicine: namely, compassion, integrity, wisdom, and other virtues that are the foundation of the trust that is essential in the doctor-patient relationship.

Students whose professional identity has been guided by the study of literature should be able to:

- Consider multiple perspectives about what it means to be a doctor and a patient
- Think critically about the profession of medicine
- Comment insightfully about how the dyadic doctor-patient relationship is situated within larger societal dynamics and discourses
- Engage in reflective analysis of professional and ethical dilemmas
- Respond appropriately to various emotions that arise in themselves and their patients and families in response to diagnosis and treatment
- Develop a deep understanding of how culture shapes differences in communication

It is noteworthy that in the aforementioned study, a "willingness to be different" was reported as a prominent unused skill, suggesting that students need to take responsibility for their own learning regardless of criteria set by medical school admission committees. Physicians who found that their college educations fostered willingness to be different tended to choose less typical medical careers, potentially contributing to a more diverse physician workforce.

There are so many important works of literature for medical students to become familiar with. Here are ten of my personal favorites:

1. ***The House of God*** by Samuel Shem: This iconic novel provides a stark look at the realities of medical training, offering a critical perspective that encourages medical professionals to maintain compassion and empathy.

2. ***Being Mortal: Medicine and What Matters in the End*** by Atul Gawande: This book delves into the challenges of aging and death, discussing how medicine can not only improve life but also the process of its ending.

3. ***The Man Who Mistook His Wife for a Hat*** by Oliver Sacks: This collection of case histories of neurological disorders offers a compassionate and insightful look into the human mind and spirit. (***Seeing Voices: A Journey into the World of the Deaf***, also by Sacks, is a good alternative.)

4. ***The Spirit Catches You and You Fall Down*** by Anne Fadiman: This book explores the clash between a small county hospital in California and a refugee family from Laos over the care of a Hmong child diagnosed with severe epilepsy.

5. ***When Breath Becomes Air*** by Paul Kalanithi: Written by a neurosurgeon diagnosed with stage IV lung cancer, this posthumously published memoir explores the nature of life and death, doctor and patient, and the relationship between health and identity.

6. ***The Death of Ivan Ilyich*** by Leo Tolstoy: This classic novella depicts a man's struggle with mortality, offering a profound exploration of the human experience of death and dying.

7. ***The Emperor of All Maladies: A Biography of Cancer*** by Siddhartha Mukherjee: This Pulitzer Prize-winning book provides a comprehensive history of cancer, its treatments, and the ongoing search for a cure.

8. ***What Doctors Feel: How Emotions Affect the Practice of Medicine*** by Danielle Ofri. This book uses the author's rich personal and clinical vignettes to dissect the hidden emotional responses of physicians and show how these directly influence patients and treatment.

9. ***My Own Country: A Doctor's Story of a Town and Its People in the Age of Aids*** by Abraham Verghese. A heart-rending and evocative account of the early days of the AIDS epidemic, with

tales of human suffering and endurance, and how a physician came to love a corner of Appalachia. (Anything written by Verghese is a good alternative.)

10. ***In Shock: My Journey from Death to Recovery and the Redemptive Power of Hope*** by Rana Awdish. By surviving a catastrophic medical event during pregnancy and countless complications, a critical care specialist is able to showcase the tremendous power of hope in the healing process.

These and many other works of literature can provide medical students with valuable insights into the human aspects of medicine beyond what they learn through science courses, textbooks, and clinical practice. Stories impart communication skills and a sensitive appreciation of the multiple dimensions of practice. Above all, reading stimulates the development of students' personal values and an enduring sense of wonder at embodied human nature.

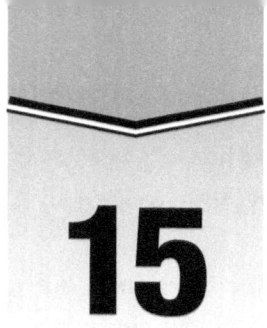

15

Medical School Applicants do not Need to "Check" a Box to Succeed

Academic excellence, personal character, and
lived experience should be sufficient.

Medical pundits are predicting that the U.S. Supreme Court ruling striking down race-conscious admissions will have dire consequences for medical schools and the composition of the physician workforce.

The concern is that the high court's decision to restrict public and private higher education institutions from considering an applicant's race or ethnicity in admission decisions will negatively impact medical schools' diversity and the nature of future physicians.

The fear is that gains made over the past few years in achieving gender, racial, and ethnic minority representation among physicians will suffer and possibly be erased, especially as legacy admissions continue to disproportionately favor white applicants over minority ones.

Few in medicine would argue the need for medical schools to recruit more students and hire more faculty that reflect the diversity of the American population. Black, Latino, and Native American residents make up 30% of the population, but just under 9% of practicing physicians. Although I am concerned about the possible negative consequences of the Supreme Court's ruling, I do not foresee a setback to ongoing efforts to diversify medicine and improve care. Here are my reasons:

1. **Race is already known prior to admission.** A medical school applicant's race is plainly visible to admissions officers who conduct interviews, whether face-to-face or by video. Even in applicants who are not selected for interviews, many elements pertaining to their identity, including race and ethnicity, can be inferred from their applications, sometimes from their names and often through self-revelatory essays. The point is racial characteristics do not have to be disclosed on an application in order for members of the admission committee to be aware of them.

2. **Medical school admissions committees are diversifying.** While it is true that historically the composition of admissions committees has maintained a white status quo, there is increasing diversity among faculty participating on admissions committees. This will likely lead to greater diversity, equity, and inclusion (DEI) among matriculating students.

3. **Community members sit on admissions committees.** Admissions officers are placing greater emphasis on how medical students connect with the community around them. At some medical schools, community members are involved in interviewing prospective medical students, and they have a vote on the school's admissions committee. Medical schools are thus in a unique position to reverse racial disparities in the profession by attracting medical students who want to work closely with the community.

4. **Internal influences, such as explicit – or, more often, implicit – biases are being acknowledged and uprooted from standing committee operations.** Implicit bias is a major factor responsible for health care disparities, and it prevents faculty and administrators from considering diversity as a needed

health intervention. However, after decades-long calls for increasing racial and ethnic diversity in the medical profession, the message finally seems to be getting through. The number of Black, Hispanic, and women applicants and enrollees continued to increase at U.S. medical schools in the 2022-23 academic year, according to the Association of American Medical Colleges. And women now outnumber men entering medical school.

5. **DEI initiatives are here to stay.** There is probably no more pressing initiative today than to increase racial and ethnic diversity across health care institutions by including members of Black or African American, Hispanic or Latino, and Indigenous groups. DEI goals and objectives have filtered down to students, faculty, and admissions committees who, in turn, have developed strategies to eliminate barriers to the advancement of diversity in medical school admissions. Medical leaders' continued removal of inequitable structures and implementation of process changes is a critical step toward achieving racial justice.

I'm optimistic (maybe overly optimistic) that checking a box that identifies one's racial and ethnic origins may no longer be necessary to further our interest in increasing the diversity of the physician workforce – it clearly is no longer constitutionally permissible. Without the identification of race, what, then, matters most in gaining admission to medical school? What are the factors that really count and will persuade a hypothetically colorblind medical school admissions committee to accept a student? The short answer is a triumvirate of core competencies – academic excellence, personal character, and lived experience. I believe these will become the new drivers of admission to medical school.

Given the ever-increasing demand for medical careers and the limited number of openings in medical schools, students must demonstrate outstanding scholastic achievement in the physical sciences, social sciences, and humanities. They must parlay this knowledge into the Medical College Admission Test (MCAT) so that the combination of their MCAT scores and overall grade point average (GPA) is compelling and demonstrates an ability to master a wide range of subjects considered a prerequisite for undertaking the vicissitudes of medical school. There are no hard cut-offs in terms of MCAT and GPA scores, but the numbers usually have to sing to admissions officers in order to be granted an interview.

No singular character type portends success in medical school and beyond, just as no specific set of attributes defines a great leader. But what is important is that students demonstrate that they have a well-developed sense of identity and character. Character comes across in the content of primary and secondary essays and personal interviews. Students who are sure of themselves, write with conviction, make good eye contact, shake hands firmly, and readily connect with people surely will stand apart from the competition. Faculty also pay close attention to students' nonverbal behavior and how they carry and conduct themselves during the interview. Successful applicants will have an altruistic sense of purpose and genuine desire to be leaders and change agents in the health professions field.

Most pre-med advisors tell medical students to gain experience in the medical field prior to applying to medical school. While this may be helpful, I'm convinced that non-medical jobs and other types of experience listed on students' resumes will count as much, if not more, than brief forays in a research lab or hospital. In my case, it was working as a beer vendor at a major league baseball park. In the case of a colleague, it was working as a jack-of-all-trades in a restaurant. There are infinite jobs and experiences outside of medicine that students can use to their advantage on essays and in interviews. Many applicants today have great diversity of experience partly due to the increased popularity of gap years.

A Black medical student transitioning into his fourth year asked me for advice. The student was tasked with describing his three most important characteristics. The medical school dean wanted to include this information in a letter to support the students' application to residency programs. The student wrote three brief paragraphs about himself, but he failed to specify the nature of the characteristics that distinguished him, which were 1) resiliency, 2) role model and educator, and 3) crusader for overcoming health disparities.

I'm sure this student will match at their first-choice program. Checking a residency application box is meaningless for someone with his talent.

16

How to (Legally) Diversify the Healthcare Workforce

Alternative approaches are key following the SCOTUS ruling on race-based admissions

The American Medical Association (AMA) has long recognized the benefits of a diverse student population in classrooms and exam rooms. Thus, it was no surprise that following the Supreme Court of the United States' (SCOTUS) decisions to virtually ban race and ethnicity as factors for admitting students to colleges and universities, several medical schools and professional organizations announced their continued commitment to diversifying the healthcare workforce: The John A. Burns School of Medicine (JABSOM) at the University of Hawaii, the Association of American Medical Colleges (AAMC), and the Accreditation Council for Graduate Medical Education (ACGME), to name a few.

To determine the potential impact of the SCOTUS ruling on medical schools' selection process, the *Philadelphia Inquirer* (August 6, 2023) interviewed two deans at Cooper Medical School of Rowan University and the former admissions director at Thomas Jefferson's Sidney Kimmel Medical College – two of seven medical schools in the Philadelphia area. The consensus was that schools might end up enrolling fewer students from underrepresented populations – a fact already borne out by research in states that have previously eliminated race and ethnicity from consideration in admissions. However, the officials hinted that there may be ways to overcome the new colorblind requirement enacted by SCOTUS, sharing the same sentiments as the AMA, AAMC, and ACGME.

For example, during a webinar with medical school leaders, David Skorton, MD, CEO of the AAMC said: "Nothing in the Supreme Court decision on race conscious admissions compels us to deviate from our mission or deviate from our goals of diversifying the healthcare workforce." The AAMC has outlined specific strategies that it hopes will permit medical schools to continue to diversify while complying with the SCOTUS ruling.

Chief among those strategies is what the AAMC calls a "holistic review," an alternate way of assessing an applicant's capabilities by considering their experiences, attributes, and academic metrics in combination with consideration of how the applicant will contribute to the school's mission, goals, and learning environment. In addition, the AAMC suggests developing "pathways to health professions" in K-12 schools by engaging community educators, administrators, and learners, and equipping underrepresented young people with healthcare competencies.

The University of Pennsylvania Perelman School of Medicine in Philadelphia and the University of Chicago Pritzker School of Medicine are among an increasing number of medical schools heavily invested in attracting a more diverse pool of applicants by establishing "pipeline programs" – efforts to expose disadvantaged students to the medical professions in middle school and high school. The earlier in the educational curriculum the better, according to Reynold Verret, PhD, president of Xavier University in New Orleans, the only historically Black catholic university in the U.S. Verret was quoted in *JAMA* as saying: "The genius of America is in the second or third grade right now." However, he noted, educational disparities in K-12 schools persist decades after desegregation.

Of course, there is no reason not to extend relationship building to diverse undergraduate institutions and community-based organizations. Medical students themselves can fulfill this role by serving as school ambassadors and reaching out to specific populations and encouraging them to apply to medical school, mentoring individuals along the way.

As discussed in the previous essay, in lieu of a "check list" that ticks off an applicants' race and ethnicity, the AAMC recommends paying close attention to application essays, which often contain content relevant to students' lived experiences and may include experiences or perspectives related to the applicant's race and ethnic background. Certain desirable features may be evident in students' essays, such as whether the student:

- Grew up in a medically underserved area
- Demonstrates eagerness to engage with medically underserved populations
- Looks forward to studying health inequities
- Speaks multiple languages
- Is a first-generation college graduate

Other strategies and tools that can be utilized can be found in the ACGME Equity Matters Equity Practice Toolkit, a learning experience "designed to empower stakeholders with the tools necessary to achieve or enhance cultures of equity." The focus of this program is "how" to achieve and maintain equitable cultures with specific instruction in "acting to dismantle racism" and dealing with implicit bias.

Another tool used to diversify medical school classes is the socioeconomic disadvantage scale. University of California Davis Medical School, ranked #3 in 2023 in diversity by *U.S. News & World Report*, gives every applicant a score from 0 to 100 that considers the applicant's family income, parental education, whether applicants come from an underserved area, whether they help support their families, and other life circumstances. Admissions decisions are based on that score, combined with the usual portfolio of grades, test scores, recommendations, essays, and interviews.

Fostering diversity in healthcare leads to innumerable benefits. Attracting and enrolling more diverse students changes the composition of the physician workforce, often resulting in improved health outcomes. By diversifying, schools may be able to graduate students more willing to practice in underserved communities. To the extent that healthcare providers can reflect the demographics and diversity of their communities, patients will feel understood and better represented. Diversity in healthcare enhances the ability to innovate by gaining a variety of perspectives, a particularly important advantage in conducting research and implementing population health management programs. Solutions and ongoing efforts to improve physician workforce diversity are imperative.

17

The Graduation Speech I've Longed to Give

By invitation only.

I've been blessed to be able to attend the "white coat" ceremonies of two of my children – one is a physician and the other is a physician assistant. There were no white coat ceremonies in my era.

White coat ceremonies proliferated around the turn of the century, a rite of passage emphasizing a first-year medical student's commitment to demonstrate scientific proficiency, act professionally, earn the trust of patients and provide compassionate care. The ceremonial cloaking of medical students in white coats, as opposed to the original black garb worn by physicians, symbolizes cleanliness and purity associated with the era of antisepsis ushered in by Joseph Lister in the late 19th century. The ceremony has expanded to other health-related fields in recent years.

Attending my children's white coat ceremonies started me thinking about what my advice would be to up-and-coming physicians. It's a speech I've longed to make, but one I've never been asked to give. The speakers at white-coat ceremonies are featured by invitation only.

My main message to medical students would be to recognize that the fates of patients is beyond their control, so they should not blame themselves for bad outcomes; they should support each other through difficult and trying times and seek help if they become emotionally overwhelmed. Unwell medical students, like unwell physicians in practice, tend to lose their professional ideals, provide suboptimal care to patients, and have less successful careers than their healthier counterparts.

I would ask medical schools to ensure professional counseling is available for the approximately 50% of students who will burn out in medical school, the 15% who will become depressed and especially the 5% to 10% who will contemplate suicide. Too many struggling students (and physicians) manage to stay under the radar, so I need to tell them there is no shame in admitting to feelings of hopelessness and seeking help for anxiety and depression. Any traumatic experience can have immediate and lasting psychological effects, and medical education is no exception.

After the suicide deaths of two newly minted doctors in New York City within days of each other in August 2014, at a time when many white coat ceremonies were occurring in medical schools across the United States, well-known physician and author Danielle Ofri, MD, PhD, pleaded to students that they do not succumb to the "tyranny of medicine."

She commented, "Medical students are asked to absorb an immense body of knowledge. Prima facie, this is a seemingly reasonable request of our doctors-to-be. But the number of facts is larger than any human being can realistically acquire, and is ever expanding. Yet we act as though this perfection of knowledge is a realistic possibility. No wonder nearly every student feels like an imposter during his or her training."

I would inform the audience that imposter syndrome is a psychological construct characterized by the persistent belief that one's success is undeserved rather than due to personal effort, skill and ability. Family and friends may think imposter syndrome is not applicable to their loved ones, but the fact is a survey of more than 3,000 physicians showed that nearly one in four doctors across the career spectrum reported feeling like an imposter. The study's findings also suggested that imposter syndrome can develop during medical school and residency and continue beyond training (essay 22), and the greater the identification with an imposter the higher the prevalence of suicidal ideation.

It should not be lost upon anyone that physicians have the highest suicide rates of any professional groups. Approximate one physician per day dies by suicide in the Unites States. Lorna Breen, MD, and several other physicians like her who practiced on the front-lines of the COVID pandemic were victims of suicide. The Doctor Lorna Breen Heroes' Foundation was established to honor her memory and to fight for the professional and emotional well-being of health workers.

When these now-energized medical students eventually become disillusioned and question why they chose medicine as a profession, I want to tell them to look forward to the "human moments" in practice – taking care of people in their most vulnerable states and becoming somewhat vulnerable in the process, but not so vulnerable that they would not ask for help, if needed. They should seek out other students and faculty whom they can trust and can be vulnerable with, meeting with them at regular intervals to discuss the ups and downs of medical school. We must cultivate a professional environment that allows medical students and trainees to better support each other.

Harvard Medical School professor and quality expert Donald M. Berwick, MD, stated to the 2010 graduates of Yale Medical School: "Those who suffer need you to be something more than a doctor; they need you to be a healer. And to become a healer, you must do something even more difficult than putting your white coat on. You must take your white coat off." To which I would add: work on improving your self-valuation, reduce your perfectionistic tendencies and foster a growth mindset.

Although physicians often do heroic things, we are humans and are subject to normal human limitations. We sometimes forget we are human when we wear our white coats. Keep in mind that white coats bear no resemblance to Superman's cape – and human's don't fly!

I will remind the distinguished faculty attending the ceremony that not all medical students who graduate will remain in practice or even enter the practice of medicine. Some, like me, will lean toward industry and non-traditional medical careers. They need to be nurtured and feel welcomed at medical school. They are not traitors to the profession. Quite the opposite. Students enrolled in dual-degreed MD-(DO)/MBA programs will provide new healthcare perspectives. They will not abandon their professional ideals. A business curriculum integrated with a medical education at any point in one's career will produce talented leaders.

I want to inform everyone that physician leadership is critical to steer health care into the future. For physicians, in a world dominated by nonmedical administrators in hospitals and health insurance companies, medical leadership is essential for health care to continue moving toward higher quality, consistent safety and streamlined efficiency. Evidence suggests that organizations and patients benefit when physicians take on leadership roles. The best performing hospitals in the United States are led by physicians.

I realize that most students who receive their white coats will practice medicine in the traditional sense, either as primary care doctors or specialists. I want them to know that they can still be effective medical leaders as busy clinicians. In fact, medical leadership may best be rendered through what is known as "expert authority," wherein a physician's unique and extensive knowledge of diseases and therapeutics, and of human nature, serves as the basis of their authority and the platform of leading. Medical leaders succeed by communicating their vision to organizations that recognize their value, and every physician has the ability to lead.

I would reassure the class that, despite feelings of inadequacy and self-doubt they may have now, the reality is that about 90% will graduate in four years. How do I know this to be true? I did the research – as a business school project of all things! For the remaining 10% of students who do not graduate medical school, primarily personal rather than scholastic problems will cause them to change their goals.

By virtue of being accepted into medical school, each student has been deemed competent and worthy to serve the suffering. What matters most is that these young and diverse doctors-in-training are passionate about improving the quality of care for patients. A doctor can do that as a practicing physician or an industry insider.

Paraphrasing the incomparable Randy Newman ("You've Got a Friend in Me"), it doesn't matter whether you wear a white coat, a business suit, or nothing at all. You can leave your hat on.

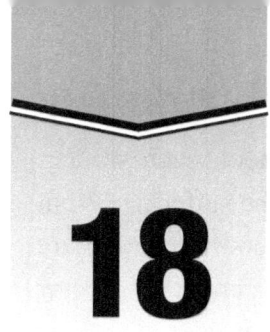

18

Bigger is Not Better in Healthcare

Mergers and acquisitions are not a recipe
for success in the medical field.

When I was a medical student and resident in Philadelphia in the late 1970s and early 1980s, there were a half-dozen medical schools within a 10-mile radius. That number was reduced to 5 in 1995 when two of the medical schools merged: The Medical College of Pennsylvania (MCP) and Hahnemann Medical College. Meanwhile, Jefferson Medical College and Jefferson Health grew by leaps and bounds, in part through acquisitions. Today, Jefferson owns 18 hospitals and a university commonly known as the Philadelphia College of Textiles and Science, renamed Philadelphia University.

While health systems may see mergers and acquisitions as the pathway to success, that's often not how the story plays out.

The union of MCP and Hahnemann was spearheaded by the late Sherif Abdelhak, the CEO of Pittsburgh-based Allegheny General Hospital. Abdelhak seized an opportunity to expand healthcare in Philadelphia much like the way Jefferson would expand – by acquiring over a dozen community hospitals. Abdelhak's empire, known as the Allegheny Health, Education, and Research Foundation, or "AHERF" for short, accumulated inordinate debt and became the largest nonprofit healthcare failure in U.S. history at the time (1998). MCP-Hahnemann emerged from the debacle as Drexel University College of Medicine.

I worked at AHERF during tumultuous times, escaping just before the organization imploded. Abdelhak warned the medical staff not to "cross" him as he went about his spending spree. (He served time in prison for misappropriating funds and later changed his last name.) Abdelhak's largesse had repercussions decades later, as years of hospital consolidation likely played a role in the closing of Hahnemann University Hospital in 2019, displacing over 500 residents and fellows in training.

Jefferson's troubles, although not as devastating as AHERF'S, also began with the acquisition of hospitals, as well as the aforementioned Philadelphia University (which was acquired in the belief that a college known for clothing design could help redesign the delivery of medical care). This novel idea has yet to bear fruit, although self-proclaimed successes of the merged schools include increased enrollment, better educational value, increased funded research, enhanced rankings, and an impressive 97% job or graduate school success rate.

From 2009 through 2016, Jefferson allegedly invested money earmarked for a medical student loan program and siphoned the profits for its own purposes rather than reinvest them in the loan program — an allegation that Jefferson denies. (The loans provided favorable terms to students who agreed to work as primary care physicians for 10 years after completing their medical degrees.) Abdelhak did something similar: He raided endowed funds to prop up AHERF's operations (he pleaded no contest to charges).

Jefferson cutting about 1% of its workforce of more than 40,000 employees in 2023 as part of an effort to trim financial losses from decreased patient volumes and double-digit increases to costs. The health system also suffered its second credit downgrade from Moody's since it began its significant expansion. Jefferson's relatively new CEO appeared to blame the previous CEO and administration for the current state of affairs, saying, "One of the reasons we are at an inflection point now is that we have never rationalized the size of our workforce through four significant mergers." Jefferson finished its

2023 fiscal year with a $231 million operating loss, excluding gains from the sales of businesses.

Jefferson seemed to follow the same playbook as AHERF, especially in its rapid expansion and alleged misuse of funds. You would have thought that Jefferson learned a lesson from the MCP-Hahnemann merger and buyout of Philadelphia hospitals.

The story is not unique to Jefferson, however. In fact, financial hardship is a tale told by many hospitals and academic medical centers and is further proof that exponentially mounting medical costs are unsustainable, if not incomprehensible, as pointed out by *Time* magazine 10 years ago.

Healthcare was never meant to be profitable. The hundreds of hospitals and health systems that have closed their doors in the past 2 decades are a tribute to that fact. In 2022 alone there were 46 healthcare bankruptcies with liabilities of $10 million or more, and the number will likely continue to rise in 2023. Solvency is not easy to maintain given unstable market conditions and higher costs for labor, pharmaceuticals, and other supplies. In addition, hospitals nationwide are grappling with a shift toward outpatient services as improvements in technology make same-day surgery and other procedures more feasible.

A single-payor system is often touted as a solution to runaway costs, but as we all know, there are many issues associated with giving the government sole control of healthcare. Rationing care is frequently discussed in the context of spiraling healthcare costs. However, we already ration care implicitly; doing so explicitly opens up a hornet's nest of ethical concerns.

I was fortunate to hear the late Princeton economist Uwe Reinhardt speak at a conference. He summed up the situation succinctly. He asked the audience to imagine an equilateral triangle with the three points of the triangle labeled as: costs, quality, and access. The problem, he said, is that we can only achieve two of the points as healthcare goals and the third must be sacrificed. For example, if we want to build a health system that provides easy access and top-notch care, costs will skyrocket. If we want the system to provide excellent quality and keep costs low, we will have to deny access to the sickest patients. Reinhardt joked that access is an elusive concept. Everyone has "access" to a Mercedes Benz, he said.

Reinhardt then asked, "What is the most expensive piece of medical equipment?" Those in attendance guessed MRIs, CT scanners, and other plausible answers. Reinhardt shook his head, then reached inside his jacket, pulled out a pen and held it high in the air for everyone to see. Individuals chuckled, suddenly aware and silently knowing that doctors' prescriptions and orders – many written strictly for defensive reasons – are among the key drivers of costs and do not necessarily lead to improved outcomes.

The conference that Reinhardt spoke at was held in the 1990s. The truth is, no one has come up with an answer to the problem of soaring healthcare costs to this day. But at least we know that bigger is not better.

19

Never Ask Me to Be a Medical Expert Witness (Again)

"Let us rely on evidenced medicine to pick the best drug when we have a choice, but not to tell us that being human and collaborating in the richness of life has no value."
—Lewis Mehl-Madrona, MD, PhD

Once, I agreed to be an expert witness. Never again! Not because I was grilled on the witness stand for several hours. Not because my qualifications were questioned. And certainly not because I was compensated poorly for my time. Rather, I don't ever want to have to defend our profession's great tradition steeped in the "art" of medicine.

A little over a decade ago, I was hired on behalf of a patient's attorney who was suing an insurance company for "bad faith" decision-making for denying the patient what I and other physicians believed was medically necessary treatment. The lawyer representing the insurance company confronted me on the stand.

"Dr. Lazarus," he belted out, "are you familiar with this textbook?" The lawyer practically heaved *Harrison's Principles of Internal Medicine* at me, further questioning whether I was familiar with the tenets of evidenced-based medicine. I have lived by those principles my entire career, I told him, but I remained silent about the real truth: the fact that "textbooks tell lies."

"Textbooks tell lies" is a phrase I've never forgotten after reading Viktor Frankl's *Man's Search for Meaning* (essay 12). Frankl and other physicians at Auschwitz concentration camp quickly learned that the information contained in medical textbooks was irrelevant to their plight, i.e., the brutal conditions their bodies and minds were required to endure. Who could have predicted the need for treatments for the myriad illnesses resulting from the unimaginable inhumanity prisoners were subjected to? And conversely, no medical textbooks of that era anticipated the surprising resiliency of some prisoners in the face of famine, torture, and disease. "Resiliency" wasn't even a concept in the early to mid-1940s.

As someone who embraced and practiced evidenced-based medicine long before the term was coined, testifying about the sanctity of the art of medicine was an interesting turn of events because I had to find it within myself to tell the lawyer how compassion and caring should have factored into the insurance company's decision. I had to channel Viktor Frankl.

My opening pitch involved telling the insurance company's lawyer that there's much more to practice than what textbooks and journal articles teach us. However, the attorney tried to shut me down, implying I was not familiar with the concept of evidenced-based medicine. He actually asked the judge to excuse me, claiming that I did not qualify as an "expert."

The judge had the good sense to let me testify, and testify I did! I explained that the art of medicine entails understanding patients' histories – where they've been and how they got here – and listening to their stories, in many instances stories of grief and destitution. To practice the art of medicine means that you know your patients inside-out, including social and psychological issues impacting their health. You know their occupation, who they are close to, and what their living situation is like. When you're a psychiatrist, you know them even more deeply. Who do they love? Who do they argue with? Who do they hold a grudge against and regret not making amends? Textbooks and journal articles do not steer you in that direction, I said to the attorney.

The lawyer objected to my testimony as being "non-responsive," but I was on a roll, and the judge held up his hand like a stop sign to the attorney and let me proceed. The art of medicine goes beyond mere knowledge obtained from double-blinded placebo-controlled studies, I continued. It requires treating the patient as a whole person, not just their illness. This includes taking into consideration their mental and emotional health, lifestyle, and personal circumstances. It demands treating patients with empathy and concern. Understanding and acknowledging a patient's feelings can greatly improve their healthcare experience and can positively influence their health outcomes. Doctors have to discover the essence of their patients' existence on their own and not through some textbook, I concluded.

The insurance company doctors who denied care to this patient knew nothing about him other than that he had condition "X" and his physician was requesting treatment "Y," which the insurance doctors considered "not medically necessary." They did not even weigh the fact that, despite the patient's current therapy, he was not responding to it and was becoming progressively blind.

Such callous decision making and patient neglect, I argued, was tantamount to practicing medicine in bad faith. My argument was a stretch because legally "bad faith" generally refers to intentional dishonest behavior or misleading actions that result in harm or potential harm, and that was not entirely evident here since the insurance company physicians were simply relying on a set of guidelines, misguided though they were. Nevertheless, the judge was sympathetic and he essentially forced the insurance company into a settlement.

The art of medicine and the science of medicine are two fundamental aspects of healthcare. They represent different but complementary approaches to patient care. The science of medicine aims to provide objective, evidence-based solutions to health problems. It provides the tools and knowledge necessary to diagnose and treat diseases.

The art of medicine, on the other hand, refers to the more subjective and personal aspect of healthcare. It involves understanding the patient as an individual, empathizing with their experiences, and building a therapeutic relationship. The art of medicine ensures that broad knowledge of the patient is applied in a compassionate and culturally competent manner. Both the art and science of medicine are necessary for effective medical practice.

I don't have anything against lawyers. I just wish more of them would read *Man's Search for Meaning.*

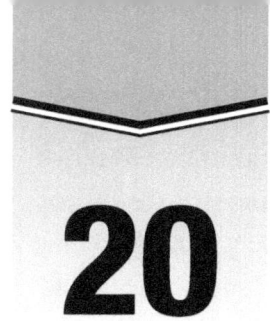

20

Let's Break a Bad Habit: Over Relying on Outcomes

"Medicine is a science of uncertainty and an art of probability."
—Sir William Osler

A colleague told me a story about his monthly nature drives with his mother who resides in a retirement center and suffers vascular dementia. Yet she remains lucid enough to have relatively normal conversations and enjoy the scenery when not complaining about the staff stealing her belongings.

"Is there an outcome to these adventures," my colleague asks? Must there be?

He then answers his own question in the negative and reflects: "These visits are to spend time with my mother while giving my siblings a bit of a break, and to get her out of her environment."

I agree with my colleague. If there is one bad habit that we have acquired in practice it is this: we are obsessed with outcomes.

I can already hear the medical pundits pushing back. Outcomes are critical in determining the effectiveness of treatments, interventions, and healthcare strategies, they will tell me. Outcomes serve as quantifiable evidence of the success or failure of medical practices. They are integral to practice guidelines, policies, and research. And so forth.

I do not dispute that medicine is fundamentally a field dedicated to improving health and saving lives, and that's why we are laser focused on outcomes. The problem is that medicine seems to be exclusively fixated on the scientific foundation of outcomes to the neglect of its humanistic dimensions. Concentrating solely on outcomes can lead to an overemphasis on data and facts, often neglecting the qualitative aspects of patient care such as patient satisfaction, comfort, and overall well-being.

An overemphasis on outcomes can lead to a one-size-fits-all approach, which may not be suitable or effective for all patients. Patients have distinctive needs and require individualized treatment plans. Outcomes are population-based and not necessarily geared to the special needs of each patient. When patients feel neglected, several consequences can occur, including emotional distress, decreased trust in healthcare providers, and harm to the doctor-patient relationship.

Outcomes focus on a limited set of measurable and quantifiable results, such as lab results or survival rates. This narrow focus can overlook other important determinants of patient health and wellness, such as emotional and spiritual well-being, social relationships, and the ability to engage in activities of daily living and other activities necessary for independent living, so-called instrumental activities of daily living.

The failure to achieve long-term health and wellness goals may result from relying on outcomes that are short sighted or only measured for a brief period. This is a common occurrence in the pharmaceutical industry, where most clinical trials designed for initial FDA approval last months rather than years. Yet many medical conditions are chronic and require long-term therapy, leaving clinicians in the dark to gather additional information based on their experience, that of their colleagues, and post-marketing surveillance and risk assessment programs to identify adverse events that did not appear during the drug approval process. It's telling that about a third of the drugs the FDA approved between 2001 and 2010 were involved in some kind of safety event after reaching the market, according to a study published in *JAMA*.

And what happens when outcomes are linked to the wrong variables or, worse yet, tied to financial incentives. It's simply unethical to design outcomes that are not in the best interest of patients and instead profit drug companies or physicians or healthcare institutions. This could lead to over-treatment or unnecessary procedures.

Additional ethical concerns are raised by using outcomes to guide treatment, such as discrimination against patients with poor prognoses, or prioritizing patients who are likely to have better outcomes. One of the most egregious instances of outcome-based discrimination was the use of an incorrect method for determining estimated glomerular filtration rate (eGFR) in Blacks that caused them to seem healthier than they really were. As a result, hospitals nationwide had to notify thousands of Black people with kidney disease of the error, which was caused by an unnecessary modifier in calculating their eGFR, and advance them on transplant waiting lists.

Outcomes, even if designed appropriately, can be misinterpreted, leading to incorrect treatment decisions. For example, a temporary improvement in symptoms may be mistaken for a cure, leading to premature termination of treatment. One of the most common mistakes in my field (psychiatry) is quite the opposite: attributing agitation to an exacerbation of the underlying psychiatric disorder when, in fact, agitation is a side effect of a patient's medication. Increasing the offending psychiatric medication or adding another drug to combat the "agitation" only compounds the situation.

There may be potential risks or side effects associated with certain treatments that could outweigh the benefits, especially if the treatment is aggressive or invasive. If the focus is solely on outcomes, these risks may be overlooked. Obtaining informed consent from patients may not address the risks given the complexity of the informed consent process and detailed level of information and understanding required to enable an informed decision.

We cannot achieve the best results for our patients by relying solely on measurable outcomes. We must also take into consideration the qualitative and interpersonal aspects of medical practice that are vital to patient care but cannot be precisely measured or quantified, like empathy, communication, trust, and understanding. All are crucial for achieving the best outcomes and providing effective healthcare. Our obsession with only the quantifiable aspects of outcomes is a bad habit. Let's break it.

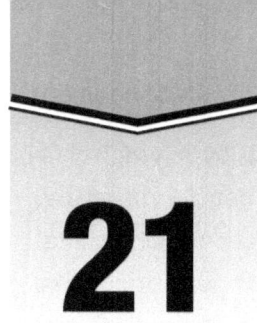

21

Memoirs of a "Recovering" Peer Reviewer

An insider's perspective.

In theory, the application of evidenced-based guidelines assists in reducing unwarranted variation in clinical practice and improving the quality and cost of care. Guideline developers, health plans, and their benefit managers contend that utilization management programs based on medically proven guidelines will transform the health of our communities, one person at a time.

Utilizing the services of physician (and nurse) advisers, guidelines are deployed in the medical review of complex, controversial, unusual, new, or experimental medical services involving proposed surgery, imaging, pharmaceuticals, devices, and various procedures. The length and level of service – for example, hospital, skilled nursing facility, outpatient treatment, and the like – are also subject to review. All this activity falls under the umbrella of utilization review (UR).

UR companies cannot exist without physician advisers. It is generally accepted, and in some instances mandated, that only a physician can deny medical services (technically, medical benefits). And therein lies the rub. Most practicing physicians detest being subjected to UR procedures – completing forms and responding to time-consuming peer reviews. An American Medical Association (AMA) survey found that, on average, physicians and their staff spend 13 hours per week (nearly 2 business days) completing prior authorization requests, which represent only a subset of UR functions.

No one knows the number of U.S. physicians working for utilization management organizations, but it is becoming increasingly popular because companies offer flexible hours and remote working opportunities. The work can be full time or as a contractor, leaving time to continue to see patients.

I used to believe strongly in the importance of UR and the tenets of utilization management – increased quality and decreased costs. I even worked for a few organizations earlier in my career. I left because I could no longer support the premise that managed care was better than care as usual, and because I questioned my right to tell another doctor how to practice medicine. The more I sympathized with my colleague on the other end of the telephone line, the more I tried to help them fulfill their request for services for their patient, regardless of the UR criteria.

One doctor thanked me for helping him document the clinical rationale necessary to extend time in the hospital for his patient. He called me an industry "insider." He said it was meant as a "compliment" because he was amazed I still cared about patients. This doctor's "compliment" insinuated he had written me off as a healer. I believe that most individuals who become doctors do so with a deep desire to help people heal. Yet, in my case, my purpose had become lost upon my colleague, and perhaps myself as well.

Another issue that plagued me was my psychiatric training, which qualified me to review mainly patients with psychiatric and substance use disorders. Nowadays, there are a host of companies contracted by payers to conduct specialty reviews in diverse areas ranging from behavioral health to orthopedic and spinal surgery to oncology treatment.

Shouldn't physicians who sub-specialize in a particular area of medicine be reviewed by equally qualified physicians? Matched specialty review has become a highly controversial topic. Specialty matches are usually required upon appeal of an adverse medical determination, but not for the first level of review. Still, I doubt that a cardiothoracic surgeon would have wanted me denying – or even approving – her proposed treatment.

Discussions with treating providers to clarify clinical information caused me considerable anxiety. I cringed at the thought of having adversarial peer-to-peer calls with other physicians. I also had misgivings about HIPAA when it was enacted. Although peer review conducted through the proper channels falls into the exception for healthcare operations, common pitfalls exist that may expose physicians to HIPAA liability.

Indeed, one physician challenged my authority to conduct peer review. Nevertheless, he complied with my request for clinical information. Subsequently, he filed an ethics complaint with the American Psychiatric Association (APA), claiming my role as a peer reviewer was unethical because I did not have his patient's permission to discuss the case. So why did he divulge the information in the first place? I was exonerated by the APA, but the experience opened my eyes to the fury of my peers.

It is not uncommon for treating physicians to intimidate reviewing physicians by asking for their credentials and licensing information and reporting them to state medical boards. Although hospital quality assurance peer review committees operate under privilege afforded by law, the same is not true for UR activities conducted by commercial entities. To the extent that such activities are tantamount to the practice of medicine, physician advisers could face licensure sanctions – for example, if they fail to competently review the medical record, behave unprofessionally, or review a case in "bad faith," i.e., with extreme prejudice or malice, as I discussed in essay 19.

UR jobs can be rewarding for some physicians. The excitement stems, in part, from the importance and critical nature of the physician adviser role, especially in utilization management companies scaled to impact millions of patients. The role caters to individuals interested in population health. And when you add UR companies' marketing pitch – working virtually or on-site in a fast-paced environment that favors individuals who are able to learn quickly, be hands-on, handle ambiguity, and communicate effectively with people of different backgrounds and perspectives – UR jobs seem like an ideal fit for physicians seeking a career change.

Unfortunately, physicians who drink the Kool-Aid soon realize UR jobs are a dead-end. There is little opportunity for upward mobility in large healthcare organizations dominated by the "suits," where business executives value physicians for their ability to save the company money by denying care to patients, and where women face a significant glass ceiling to advancement.

I believe fewer physicians would work for UR companies if they fully understood the burden of UR on practicing physicians and their patients and employers. The aforementioned AMA survey found that prior authorization requirements substantially delay treatment, force physicians to abandon treatment, and negatively impact clinical outcomes and work performance. I recommend physicians think twice about drinking the beverage they're served.

22

Practicing Medicine with Conviction

Acres of diamonds.

What does it take for physicians to practice with conviction – to practice medicine with a sense of confidence and commitment, passionate about your work? What factors allow medical students to enter the resident pool each July and turn their timidness into poise? How do you learn to stand by your medical convictions and base your decision making on a deep understanding of the patient combined with the latest evidence-based practices? Here are a few thoughts that come to mind.

First and foremost is continuous learning. You can practice with conviction by being well-informed and up-to-date about the latest medical advancements, research, and practices. This includes attending medical conferences, participating in professional development activities, and reading the latest medical journals.

I suggest you read (or skim) at least one major medical journal each week, like the *New England Journal of Medicine* or the *Journal of the American Medical Association* (*JAMA*), and two highly regarded journals in your specialty. A daily or weekly online newsfeed is also useful. Why not listen to a podcast on your way into work?

The pace of medical advancements can sometimes be overwhelming, making it challenging for you to stay updated. You must find the time to read, however, because reading bolsters your confidence and strengthens your commitment. During rounds, I frequently distributed articles relevant to patients on our service, and I was proud to be called "Article" Lazarus by the house staff. I could always take a ribbing in the name of patient care.

The more knowledge and experience you have, the more conviction you will have in your decisions and actions. This comes from years of practice, dealing with various cases, and learning from successes and failures – and you will fail, make no mistake about it. The Institute of Medicine wrote "To Err is Human." I keep a placard in my office that reads: "I am willing to make mistakes if someone else is willing to learn from them."

Doctors with conviction are able to empathize with their patients. They understand their concerns, fears, and expectations, which helps them provide the best possible care. We must never let our empathy wane. When choosing a physician, patients value affective concern as much as, if not more than, technical competence. I am dismayed by studies showing empathy decreasing midway through medical school, before doctors are newly minted. Medical students should realize that physicians who are more attuned to the psychosocial needs of their patients are more likely to have better outcomes.

A physician practicing with conviction adheres strictly to medical ethics. This includes respecting patients' rights, maintaining confidentiality, and avoiding any form of discrimination. We are at a tipping point where the promulgation of diversity, equity and inclusiveness initiatives are beginning to eradicate barriers to treatment for minority populations while promoting a more diverse physician workforce. Diversity – or the lack of it – among medical students and physicians affects not only how care is delivered but also the ability to make clinical decisions with conviction and courage.

A nurturing environment is essential to practicing with conviction. Trainees are more capable of rising to a clinical challenge when they are respected and treated well. Our collective experience reveals that it is not a health system or long working hours that guarantees residents become excellent physicians; it's the conviction and dedication of the people within those systems and who schedule the hours.

In order to practice with conviction, certain barriers must be overcome. The most important is imposter syndrome (IS), as I discussed in essay 17. People often think of imposter syndrome as a lack of self-confidence, and although that is certainly a feature, the hallmark of IS is an internal feeling of intellectual phoniness, a persistent belief that you are really not bright and have fooled anyone who thinks otherwise. Individuals with IS are high achievers, but they doubt their accomplishments and believe they are unwarranted.

Anyone who dreads being exposed as a "fraud" cannot practice with confidence. You will be saddled with doubts and fears of failing, as well as constant anxiety. Physicians with IS may be less likely to seek help or advice from their colleagues due to fear of appearing incompetent. This can hinder communication and teamwork, which are crucial in the management of patients.

A lack of confidence can also be perceived by patients, potentially undermining their trust in doctors and the profession. The first time I was called on to perform venipuncture on a patient I was a nervous wreck. My hands were trembling. The patient was keenly aware of my insecurity and refused to allow me to draw blood. My confidence was shaken, and I shied away from performing procedures afterward.

Imposter syndrome can become a self-fulfilling prophecy because it keeps physicians from achieving their full potential. They develop an aversion to being in the spotlight and turn down leadership opportunities. For these reasons and others, discussions about IS should be integrated early into medical student and residency wellness programs and initiatives. Students deeply affected by IS, believing they are truly fakes, should seek psychotherapy.

There may be several conditions other than IS that affect physicians' commitment to practice. Prominent among them is burnout: exhaustion, cynicism, and reduced professional efficiency. Burnout clearly affects doctors' commitment and passion for their work. A major cause of burnout is chronic stress often brought on by practicing with limited resources, whether it's time, staff, equipment, or funding, which can prevent physicians from providing the best care possible, affecting their conviction. Physicians can take action to prevent burnout and seek help early when it occurs, restoring their commitment to practice.

Clinical uncertainties and treatment ambiguities can sometimes affect a physician's conviction, especially in the context of malpractice litigation. Simply the fear of litigation can make physicians practice defensive medicine rather than making decisions based solely on their professional judgment. The manner in which doctors deal with uncertainty affects their emotional well-being and ultimately their conviction to practice. Your interest in and commitment to practice will skyrocket once you learn that medicine is not always black and white and develop skills to better tolerate ambiguity. In my case, learning to cope with uncertainty required psychotherapy, as I discuss in essay 38.

Systemic pressures – pressures from insurance companies, hospital administrators, and many other parties tied to the "medical-industrial complex" – can sometimes force doctors to make decisions that they are not entirely comfortable with, thereby affecting their conviction. Moral injury resulting from the failure of health systems to protect physicians during and after COVID has made them rethink their commitment to medicine, and they are leaving in droves. Healthcare institutions should focus on administrative and climate interventions to prevent and address moral injury and secure the physician workforce.

Finally, institutions and academicians must look more carefully at their processes to make sure those creative, out-of-the-box thinkers with potential are not lost in the shuffle of medical school and early career practice.

A case in point is Katalin ("Kati") Karikó, a pioneering American-Hungarian biochemist and researcher. Karikó was rejected for a tenure track post at The University of Pennsylvania Perelman School of Medicine; she was told she was "not of faculty quality." Karikó was demoted and her pay was cut, so she left Penn and obtained a job in 2013 working for the German drugmaker BioNTech. Ten years later, Karikó and her colleague Drew Weissman, MD, PhD, won the Nobel Prize in Physiology or Medicine for their work on messenger-RNA research that paved the way for COVID-19 vaccines. However, Karikó would rather talk about how to formalize institutional support to ensure less-celebrated scholars and their work don't fall through the cracks.

I highlight Karikó's story because it's inspirational in the same vein as Russell Conwell's (1843-1925) famous "Acres of Diamonds" speech, which became the impetus for the founding of Temple University, where I graduated medical school and business school. The story tells of an African farmer who envied other farmers, not realizing his own farm contained diamonds in raw form. Each and every one of us is diamond in the rough waiting to be cultivated. Educators should never forget their obligation to students and to help them realize their full potential, carefully identifying students who may waiver in conviction and doubt their own abilities, so that these students may sparkle with further aid and instruction.

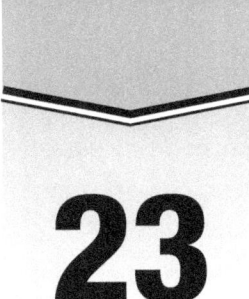

23

Reading Our Patients' Facial Expressions

Learning from Will Smith's meltdown.

As a psychiatrist, it would be unethical of me to render a diagnosis about a public figure, especially without diagnosing them. But I think it's safe to say that actor/comedian Will Smith has an anger problem. His 2022 Oscar smackdown of fellow comedian Chris Rock proves one thing: violence should never be a response to insults – or any other inciting factors – in the heat of the moment or any other time. Will Smith knows it, and so do the millions of television viewers who witnessed the assault. Yet, despite Smith's written apology to Rock and the Academy, Smith may likely believe his actions were justified.

Why do I say this? Because if you look at Smith's facial expression as he does an about-face on the stage and returns to his beloved Jada, he grins, looks upward, and appears completely satisfied with himself, maintaining a stoic appearance after the scene played out and refusing to leave the Dolby Theatre as requested by Academy officials. Smith's emotional coolness and detachment from the incident signaled self-righteousness. He was banned from future Oscar galas and associated events until 2032.

I've studied facial expressions for over 40 years, even prior to medical school, when, as an undergraduate psychology major, one of my first book purchases was Charles Darwin's *The Expression of Emotion in Man and Animals*. Darwin explained the origins of human facial expressions in the animal world and argued that facial expressions are largely innate and the same in all societies, reflecting their evolutionary and genetic rather than cultural origins. Since Darwin's time, however, evolutionary theorists have documented that much of our behavior (though perhaps not our facial expressions) is also learned and therefore the result of social factors and interactions.

Putting aside the nature-nurture controversy, facial expressions provide a compelling glimpse into people's psyches. Any expression or body language expert will tell you that facial expressions provide valuable signs for recognizing people's true emotions. Facial expressions reflect six universal emotions: surprise, fear, disgust, anger, happiness, and sadness, and they can be important clues to deceit by masking, simulating, or neutralizing emotions. A physician's ability to interpret the emotion behind a patient's facial expression makes them more adept at the practice of medicine.

Emotional awareness is just as important as emotional intelligence. But too often, we are pressed for time and ignore or inaccurately read our patients' facial expressions. The awkward positioning of computers for data entry makes it difficult to look up and see our patients. If we can't visualize them, how can we possibly understand their expressions or gather clues from other non-verbal responses? How can we judge whether their answers to critical questions belie their non-verbal behavior? In my experience, discrepancies between verbal and non-verbal behavior often surround answers to questions related to pain and mental health. Patients may paint a rosy picture of health when, in reality, they are suffering from pain, depression, or addiction.

Emojis have become a cheap and quick workaround to understanding our patients' feelings. Emojis are becoming more common in the medical setting, and some clinicians are advocating for their adoption. Doximity conducted a poll among clinicians, inquiring whether emojis should be used in a professional setting. More than two-thirds of respondents answered definitely not, or only with colleagues, but not with patients. We should not be fooled into thinking that simplistic caricatures can substitute for signs of observable distress in our patients or replace what is at the heart of the doctor-patient relationship – good eye contact, personal communication, and the ability to interpret and discuss our patients' facial expressions and non-verbal gestures.

Despite the increased use of clinical simulations in medical school, the importance of identifying emotional facial expressions remains largely overlooked in the medical curriculum. The "proof" comes from a 2021 study conducted in India where 106 medical students were shown static images of the six universal facial expressions. About half of the students misidentified negative emotions (fear, anger, etc.), whereas the recognition of positive expressions such as happiness was much better (greater than 90% accuracy). There were no significant differences between male and female medical students, but the accuracy of identifications showed significant variations with respect to the gender of the expressors (images).

The study authors concluded that the findings were "troubling [because] future doctors might have potential difficulty in picking up subtle non-verbal cues that are so important in a doctor-patient relationship and communication with the family members." Furthermore, most emotions are expressed in real practice situations with lesser intensity than static images, making their detection more difficult. Fortunately, physicians and physicians-in-training can effectively learn to recognize emotion by interpreting facial expressions through a short workshop or similar didactic program. As doctors, it is imperative that we learn to recognize and explore patients' non-verbal cues in their speech patterns, facial expressions, and body posture.

The identification of facial expressions in patients presenting with medical emergencies may be very problematic. A study found that patients with serious and sometimes life-threatening heart or lung problems tend to have less than the normal range of facial expression, particularly when it comes to registering surprise in response to certain emotional cues. The study authors speculated that underlying serious illness may make it more challenging for patients to process emotions as a healthy person would. Accurate detection of facial expressions during an emergency could be difficult yet it is of utmost importance as it could give doctors a life-saving clue.

Some of the most effective ways to assess a patient's condition don't involve a high-tech test or scan, but rather human interaction with the patient. I always remind medical students to look at the patient before they look at the computer. Many of our patients are at their breaking points, manifested in record rates of suicide attempts, opioid overdose deaths, and in verbal and physical attacks on others. We can't afford to overlook serious psychopathology by neglecting our patients' appearance. Indeed, "general appearance" is the first category addressed on a routine mental status exam.

Stress has also taken a toll on providers. We need to be aware of our own non-verbal behavior – eye contact, body position and posture, movement, facial expression, and use of voice – as these can all influence the tone and course of an office visit or consultation. Patients frequently refer to our facial expressions and other non-verbal communication to describe and evaluate their interactions with us. This is where our emotional intelligence comes into play – the ability to understand, monitor, and control our own behavior – verbal and non-verbal – towards our patients.

Will and Jada Pinkett Smith's emotions were on full display Oscar night, and understandably so. Jada's rolling of her eyes clearly signaled she was disgusted with Rock's insulting joke comparing her to G.I. Jane, a reference to Pinkett Smith's shaved head which was similar to that of Demi Moore's in the original film but was actually the result of Pinkett Smith's alopecia and not an intentional copy-cat. Will's initial laughter at the joke morphed into rage and sanctimoniousness after smacking Rock and returning to his seat. Smith should have kept his cool, talked to Rock afterward, and asked him to apologize. At the very least, Smith could have benefited from a moment of reflection or meditation and might have responded differently. We'll never know. But we know that after he struck Rock, the nature of his facial expression will always question the sincerity of his apology.

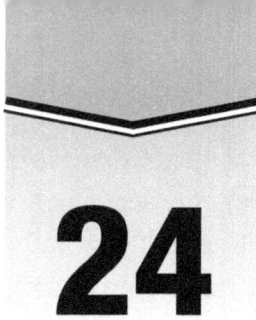

24

PTSD Due to Practice

Dear Art:

On Friday, June 11, 1982, members of the faculty convened to discuss the performance of the psychiatric residents during the last six (6) months. The following is a summation of their comments as they apply to your performance.

The faculty's reaction to your performance was uniformly excellent. There was some comment on your earlier fear of the psychotherapeutic role, but the consensus was that this has improved markedly and that you now have become more comfortable to the obvious pleasure of your faculty. There were comments about the diligence of your reading in the field and there were quotes such as "topnotch," "terrific," "a good teacher."

Art, the comments speak for themselves. We are delighted at your performance in the past year and consider you to be an outstanding resident. I am delighted with this report and look forward to your continuing in this direction in the next academic year.

Best wishes.

Sincerely yours,
[Name Withheld]
Professor and Chairman
Department of Psychiatry

I received that letter over 40 years ago, at the end of a hellish second year of residency, and finally on the upswing from depression and PTSD. Unknown to everyone except my spouse and psychiatrist, I was recovering from the effects of "vicarious" or "secondary" trauma, defined as "the destructive emotional distress resultant of an encounter with a traumatized and suffering patient or client who has suffered primary or direct trauma."

Except in my case, I did not have a close encounter with a traumatized patient, at least not technically, because I never met the patient who traumatized me.

In the spring of 1981, toward the end of my first year of residency, I was "on call" and asked to give an opinion about a patient in the emergency department (ED) who was "hearing voices." The ED resident wanted my advice about his medication, but she said it was not necessary to come to the ED to evaluate him. After assuring me over the phone that the patient was not dangerous, I suggested she increase his haloperidol dose.

The patient was discharged, but he returned to the ED several hours later following a suicide attempt – the patient had jumped out the third-story window of his boarding home. He survived the fall but sustained significant orthopedic injuries.

I blamed myself for the incident, succumbing to the moral injury of violating my personal code of excellence. "I should have seen the patient," I thought. My injury was compounded by shame and guilt, as news of what had happened quickly circulated among the house staff. I slipped into a deep depression, barely able to function.

My midyear PGY-II evaluation (December 1981) was so bad that I was placed on probation. Clearly, I was not a rising star in the eyes of the faculty, some of whom had known me since I was a medical student. My fall from grace was cemented after one of the faculty members – the individual who actually interviewed me and recommended me for medical school admission – informed me there was no way to "sugarcoat" my abysmal performance.

Psychotherapy saved my life and allowed me to complete my residency, even regaining my star status as chief resident. But I was never able to overcome the "fear of the psychotherapeutic role" referenced in my chairman's letter. Every new patient encounter heightened my anxiety. What if they were suicidal? What if they were dangerous and harmed someone? I couldn't bear the thought of being responsible for someone's actions that might result in a fatal or near-fatal outcome and cause another stain on my record.

As a form of self-therapy, I published a "coming out" article about the incident in *The Pharos* (Summer 2014), albeit 33 years after it occurred. I was humbled by the many physicians who responded to the article and shared similar experiences of vicarious traumatization.

An obstetrician-gynecologist wrote: "I, too, have a memorable patient I never saw when I was in training, and I continue to feel waves of shame and sadness over the outcome which might have been prevented if I had not gone back to sleep when the resident assured me that it was not necessary for me to see the patient."

A colleague confided that when he was a resident and moonlighting at a crisis center, he evaluated and discharged a man who went home and killed his partner. The homicide was covered by the local newspaper and television stations. My colleague escaped mention, but he was crushed by the ordeal, plagued by intrusive memories and disturbed sleep for months afterward – signs and symptoms typical of PTSD.

It is rarely appreciated that physicians who are exposed to traumatic events or trauma survivors can, themselves, become traumatized – approximately 10% to 20% develop PTSD. Surgeons and emergency medicine physicians tend to have higher rates of PTSD for obvious reasons: They treat a disproportionate number of traumatically injured patients. Psychiatrists and psychotherapists are susceptible because their patients discuss aversive details of traumatic experiences during therapy.

Physicians traumatized by unanticipated outcomes such as death; surgical complications; medical mistakes, errors, and misadventures;

and malpractice litigation may also develop PTSD. These physicians often consider themselves "innocent bystanders" to trauma. Nevertheless, the emotional impact can be severe and lasting.

One physician who wrote to me recalled how he was traumatized by a malpractice lawsuit and further traumatized when his attorney pressured him to settle it. Failing to "get his day in court," where he was certain he would be vindicated, significantly contributed to his PTSD and "emotional inability to stay in practice."

Many physicians feel they have been pushed to their limits, traumatized by a variety of practice-related stressors, not least by working in a dysfunctional health system with inadequate resources and where the threat of violence perpetuated by disgruntled patients looms large. And it's not only physicians who feel threatened – health technicians and healthcare support workers feel that way too. Witness the 85,000 Kaiser Permanente staffers who walked off the job in October 2023 demanding higher pay, increased staffing, and safer working conditions. Why shouldn't they protest for better working conditions (next essay)?

25

We Must Protest Our Moral Outrage

"We haven't had that spirit here since 1969."
— Glenn Frey/Don Felder/Don Henley
(From "Hotel California" by The Eagles)

I've finally figured out why we – physicians – are called "providers." It's not merely because we render services. In addition, our role has become a commodity, genericized and stripped of autonomy. We are no longer free to practice as we wish. We have lost the ability to take medical matters into our own hands, to control them, and to resolve them ourselves. Having lost ownership of medical practice to other people – lawyers, lawmakers, politicians, hospitals, insurance companies, licensing boards, and professional societies and organizations – decisions are made without our input or regard and certainly not in our best interest.

I guess I've known this for a long time. It's part of the reason I left practice 25 years ago at age 45 and at the height of my medical prowess and earning potential. Reading about how some physicians have recently been arbitrarily stripped of their credentials only reaffirms my decision to leave practice early rather than let the authorities chip away at it. The doctors I refer to have allegedly misinformed patients about various treatments for COVID, and they now face disciplinary action, including two physicians who have lost their American Board of Internal Medicine (ABIM) certification.

I realize some doctors need to be reined in for their outrageous behavior and remarks – for example, an Ohio physician whose license was revoked for claiming that COVID vaccines could cause people to become magnetized or create an interface with 5G towers. But they are outliers, and that's not the point I'm making here. What I am saying is that, increasingly, physicians are becoming the unjustified targets of assault on their licensure, livelihood, and constitutional rights. And the medical profession is so fragmented and subspecialized that it cannot mount a cohesive attack to fight these injustices.

One concerning issue is maintenance of certification (MOC), which is required by all specialties. Despite a decade of protest to eliminate MOC requirements, they have become more onerous, involving a substantial amount of time and money but failing to test the skill and experience of a physician. Besides, MOC content is highly redundant with continuing medical education that is a prerequisite for medical licensure in every state.

Nevertheless, ABIM stands behind its MOC program and thinks it makes physicians better doctors. The reality, according to Jay Giri, MD, an interventional cardiologist at the Hospital of the University of Pennsylvania, is that the debate lacks hard evidence and is "mostly people's opinions." Why do physicians who were recently certified need to participate in MOC? Aren't these doctors more up-to-date than physicians who were "grandfathered," i.e., allowed to retain lifetime certification before MOC existed. In theory, MOC would be more beneficial to grandfathered physicians since they are more distanced from their medical education and training.

Aaron Goodman, MD, a hematology-oncology physician at the University of California-San Diego, initiated a petition to eliminate MOC requirements for internal medicine. Over 20,000 signatures were collected, yet that represents only a fraction of the number of doctors certified by ABIM (>200,000). One can only surmise that the majority of physicians are unaware of the petition, compliant with MOC and disinterested in its broader implications for the practice of medicine, or are under the impression that attempts to overturn MOC requirements are futile.

Mark Lopatin, MD, a rheumatologist in suburban Philadelphia, postulates "that there have been so many forces exerting detrimental changes to health care that many of us have simply given up." He likens the situation to "learned helplessness," a state of apathy and depression described by the psychologist Martin Seligman in experiments with dogs who could not escape electric shocks even when given the opportunity to do so. Our inability to shake off apathy and advocate for ourselves, our patients, and our profession is what sustains the medical-industrial complex, gives corporations the upper hand, and allows them to manipulate the system for their own gain, ignoring the desires of physicians along the way.

Jordan Grumet, MD, an internal medicine physician and host of the Earn & Invest Podcast, is in agreement. He describes a type of demand apathy resulting from "tending to the insurance companies, the government, the hospital, the medical group administrators, and the electronic medical record." There's nothing left in the tank at the end of the day for our patients and ourselves, Grumet observes. Protesting is an afterthought even as we grieve the exodus of doctors from medicine and the downfall of our once proud profession.

However, protesting is not a bad idea. Lopatin said he was oblivious to the politics of medicine until he was wrongfully sued 20 years ago. Since then, he has become very active in grassroots movements and organized medicine as a strong advocate for the preservation of the patient-physician relationship. Lopatin has written numerous articles, lectured, done podcasts, and testified on subjects such as the harms of prior authorization, pharmacy benefit managers, scope creep, and, yes: MOC.

I, too, am disaffected by the loss of control over medical practice and the dissolution of our identity as healers. As I said, disillusionment with medical practice drove me away from seeing patients. Ironically, similar circumstances steered me into industry – to work as an "insider" to combat the problems thrust upon physicians by the medical bureaucracy (see essay 21).

I came out of retirement to work for an organization that provides mental health insurance and manages services for disabled and disadvantaged children and indigent adults. The company has a strong community presence and mission as well as an altruistic social agenda. I feel as though I can effect positive changes in health care delivery from the perspective of a population health medical director.

I could have taken many other routes to fight moral indignation: join pro-physician organizations, return to practice independently, and even attempt to unionize my colleagues. What matters most, I believe, is doing something about our outrage, including writing and talking about it and protesting against authorities. From Tuskegee to Tiananmen Square, social protests have sparked constructive political and policy changes by influencing the knowledge, attitudes, and behaviors of the public and organizations and institutions.

I don't consider myself an activist, but I have protested various causes from time to time. I was initiated into the art of protesting as a freshman at Boston University (BU). Then president John R. Silber invited Marines on campus to recruit students for the Vietnam War. Talk about chutzpah! I joined the picket line to prevent students from gaining access to the building where the Marines were housed. Thirty-three students were arrested that cold spring day (March 27, 1972), infamously becoming known as the "BU 33."

I was not among those arrested, but I did join many other protests as anger over the Vietnam War intensified. It seemed there was never a shortage of opportunities to join a protest in the years 1965 through 1975, a time when social and civil rights were front and center and marches, boycotts, sit-ins, and freedom summers were common. Because physicians of that era are retiring, it's up to younger generations to carry the torch. An uprising is long overdue. Perhaps a collective work stoppage would gain the nation's attention, as did the one at Kaiser Permanente, in which workers won a 21% raise over four years and secured efforts to ensure an adequate supply of new employees for the future. Next time let's include doctors in the strike.

In the iconic Eagles song Hotel California, the narrator (sung by Don Henley) calls for a bottle of wine. "We haven't had that spirit here since 1969," remarks the Captain. Hotel California has been described as an allegory for the rise and fall of the 1960s, capturing that decades' revolutionary energy, only to be extinguished by 1975. I'd like to think that the wine was maturing during the past half-century. Now it needs to be uncorked and savored – much like a revolution. We must convince people that physicians are not sheep prone to bowing before authority.

What will it take for you to join the protest and speak out against those who seek to destroy us?

26

Act Smart on Social Media

"Stupid is as stupid does."
—Forrest Gump's mama

It's understandable and even natural to want to protest the many medical irregularities and hardships plaguing practitioners today, as I discussed in the previous essay, and it's easy to channel that protest through social media outlets. However, online posts have sunk the careers of many physicians. The things that get doctors in trouble are usually caused by bad decisions and poor judgment perpetuated over TikTok, Facebook, YouTube, X (formerly Twitter) and other platforms – and there seems to be no end in sight to the misguided behavior of some physicians. Even when their actions have not been intentionally provocative or harmful, doctors' posts have received unwelcome attention from their peers, patients and medical licensing boards. It is this close scrutiny that has sealed their dooms.

Here are the 10 most common types of gaffes I've encountered online:

1. **Technical miscues**. Mark L. Tykocinski, MD, president of Thomas Jefferson University and dean of its Sidney Kimmel medical college, was a Twitter novice who used his account to "like" tweets that were critical of diversity efforts on college campuses, questioned the science of COVID-19 vaccines, and called transgender reassignment surgery "child mutilation."

Tykocinski said he "liked" the tweets in order to bookmark them for later learning. Apparently, he did not understand how 'liking' a tweet is an implied endorsement, and it caused his views on these complex issues to be questioned. Tykocinski resigned his position months afterward.

2. **Mishandling Diversity, Equity and Inclusion (DEI) Initiatives.** Howard Bauchner, MD, a pediatrician, was forced to relinquish his prestigious position as editor-in-chief of the Journal of the American Medical Association (*JAMA*) in 2021 following a controversy sparked by a *JAMA*-sponsored podcast that questioned whether structural racism existed in medicine when it was obvious that it did exist. Bauchner apologized for "lapses" that led to the publishing of the tweet and podcast, acknowledging that although he was not directly involved in the episode, he was ultimately responsible for it.

3. **Marketing unproven treatments.** William Merlino, MD, a retired New Jersey family medicine physician, was sentenced to nearly 3 years in federal prison for manufacturing and selling the toxic chemical 2,4-Dinitrophenol – better known by the name DNP – over the internet to hundreds of customers seeking to quickly lose weight. DNP is intended for industrial and agricultural use and has been banned by the FDA for human consumption since the 1930s. Federal agents shut down his operation because a British body-builder who purchased the drug from Merlino died while using it. Merlino attempted to feign a terminal illness to evade prosecution.

4. **Defying Government Agencies (DEA, IRS, etc.).** My medical school classmate, Elias Karkalas, MD, a family medicine physician practicing in suburban Philadelphia, Pennsylvania, worked part-time for an internet pharmacy company. In 2013, Karkalas was indicted by a federal grand jury in Minnesota on 38 counts of violating the Controlled Substances Act in the distribution of Fioricet to patients with headache and other

types of pain, as well as charges related to conspiracy, wire fraud, mail fraud, and introducing misbranded drugs into interstate commerce. He was able to mount a successful defense arguing that although Fioricet, a combination drug, contains butalbital, a derivative of barbituric acid, which is listed as a controlled substance (Schedule III), Fioricet, itself, was not expressly listed as a controlled substance in the *Physicians' Desk Reference* during the years he prescribed it (2005-2012). Nevertheless, Karkalas was arrested at his office, detained pretrial for 6 months, and lost his license to practice medicine for several years.

5. **Violating Existing Laws.** Despite the 1990 passage of the Native American Graves Protection and Repatriation Act, a federal law calling for the return of Indigenous human remains to descendants and tribal nations, the remains of more than 110,000 Native American, Native Hawaiian and Alaska Natives' ancestors are still held by museums, universities and federal agencies. The prestigious Mutter Museum in Philadelphia, Pennsylvania was caught in the crosshairs and has been slowly removing nearly all its violative and offending YouTube videos and many images from its website and Instagram account. However, the remains of 49 of 57 Native Americans housed by the Mutter Museum had not been made available for return by October 2023 (see essay 30). Any museum that fails to comply with the Act may be assessed a civil penalty. President and CEO Mira Irons, MD, resigned in the wake of the controversy.

6. **Livestreaming procedures**. The license of plastic surgeon Katherine Roxanne Grawe, MD, was revoked in 2023 for livestreaming operations on TikTok. Several of her patients were seriously injured allegedly due to Grawe's inattention to her patients while she was looking at the camera when filming procedures. Grawe continued to operate despite previous warnings by the Ohio medical board to protect patient privacy

on social media. Other surgeons have been reprimanded by state medical boards for inappropriately livestreaming procedures on social media and producing content that violates HIPAA.

7. **Spying on colleagues.** Boston University researchers culled snapshots of vascular surgical residents from their Facebook, Twitter, and Instagram accounts. The researchers were determined to assess whether the trainees' projected a professional image on social media. However, many readers objected to the study, and the *Journal of Vascular Surgery* retracted the article. The authors apologized for being "judgmental" and making the young surgeons feel targeted.

8. **Disseminating egregious or patently false information.** Simone Gold, MD, JD, became widely known for spreading debunked claims about COVID-19. She was sentenced to 60 days in prison – not for her unscientific and anti-vax views, however; rather, for illegally entering and remaining in the US Capitol during the January 6, 2021 insurrection. According to Gold's lawyers, the California medical board sent her a letter threatening to revoke her medical license for "an instance of misinformation." Many medical organizations have since issued statements about the harmful effects of misinformation, including the Federation of State Medical Boards, which warned that promoting misinformation could put a physician's license at risk.

9. **Posting poor quality information.** Researchers from the University of Texas Medical Branch at Galveston examined the quality of content in YouTube and TikTok videos on dissociative identity disorder (DID), a psychiatric condition characterized by the presence of 2 or more distinct personality states or an experience of possession. Only 5% of the TikTok videos were deemed "useful," and the researchers rated only about half of the YouTube videos as useful. While medical discussions offer

an opportunity for education, the threat of misinformation looms as well.

10. **Behaving unprofessionally.** In 2011, emergency medicine physician Alexandra Thran, MD, was reprimanded by the Rhode Island board of medicine for "unprofessional conduct" and fined $500 after making comments on Facebook about a patient. Thran did not mention the patient's name in the post; however, sufficient information was included that allowed others within the community to identify the patient. Thran's hospital privileges were terminated, and she was required to take a continuing education course on physician-patient confidentiality.

When Forrest Gump said "stupid is as stupid does," he meant that the actions of people, opposed to their appearance, often are an indicator of their intelligence or lack thereof. Physicians are among the brightest people on earth. Yet intelligence does not confer immunity from social media blunders.

Healthcare professionals should strive to create accurate content of high quality on social media platforms, particularly TikTok, in order to educate their peers and the public. Doctors should not sell products that are the medical equivalent of snake oil, or turn to voyeurism or writing prescriptions for unproven and illegitimate uses of medications over the internet. Any procedure that is livestreamed should be well rehearsed and done to demonstrate proper technique and technology with dignity and full informed consent of the patient. Lastly, doctors should not engage on social media platforms if they do not understand the inner-workings of the application.

NARRATIVE OF
ILLNESS & HEALING

27

A Season of Emotions:
Spring, Trauma, and Healing

Spring is an interesting time of the year for me. April 15 may actually be my favorite day, but certainly not because income taxes are due. My dad was born on April 15, but that's not the reason either.

Let me set the scene. I lived in a beautiful home in a wooded area outside Philadelphia for ten years. The area is known as the Brandywine Valley. It's the site of the Battle of Brandywine (September 11, 1777), the bloodiest and deadliest of skirmishes during the Revolutionary War. The Brandywine Valley is also home to individuals with impeccable lineage: the famous DuPont (chemicals) and Wyeth (painting) families.

Our modest one-acre home had a koi pond out front. The pond was spanned by a small bridge that served as a walkway connecting the front yard to the front door. The koi hibernated at the bottom of the pond during the cold months of December through March. An expert told me not to feed the fish during wintertime, because their metabolism was so slow that they would "implode" if they ate.

Come April 15, however, after several months of hibernation, with spring on the horizon and nature beginning to bloom, the koi were ready to surface and eat. I would stand at the apex of the bridge and dangle food pellets in their line of view. Conditioning would bring them to the pond's surface. The fish opened their mouths, waiting – no, begging – for me to drop the pellets in the water. They devoured the food. Once again it was possible to begin my ritual of daily feedings from the bridge.

Life seems to start anew each spring. It holds tremendous symbolism for renewal and regrowth. I'm reminded of the classic 1949 movie "It Happens Every Spring." The movie is about a chemist-turned-baseball pitcher who invents a compound that, when applied to the baseball, repels wood, so bats can't hit it. Thus, he is able to strike out every batter. However, the pitcher is unable to manufacture the secret sauce just when he needs it the most: during the World Series. He must rely on his own skills to win the game. And of course, he does win!

My favorite baseball movie is "Field of Dreams." I used to watch it every spring with my son. We are geographically distanced now, but we reenact some of our favorite scenes on the phone at the beginning of spring training. "Field of Dreams" is the ultimate father and son bonding movie, in my opinion. Neither of us refrains from crying at the end, when the son (Kevin Costner) asks his dad if he wants to have a catch. Such is a time-honored tradition between a father and a son, and Lord knows, my son and I have had many catches

Springtime isn't all roses. I was traumatized in the month of April when I was a psychiatric resident, in 1981, as I described in essay 24. To recapitulate, a young man attempted suicide by jumping out of the third story of his boarding home. I was blamed for the incident because I did not evaluate him in the emergency department hours prior to the suicide attempt. In truth, I was never asked to evaluate him. Still, guilt and shame set in, the primary ingredients for depression and PTSD, as I discuss in the following essay. I carried the burden of his injuries most of my career, never letting on that a fear of making mistakes was the main reason I eventually left practice. I decided to "come out" in 2014 and write about the incident. My article was warmly received. Several doctors wrote to me describing similar fates and circumstances related to medical errors falsely attributed to them.

The groundbreaking 1999 Institute of Medicine (IOM) report said "To Err is Human." The report stressed that systems are more often at fault than individuals when it comes to medical error. I felt somewhat vindicated. But the IOM report also estimated that nearly 100,000 Americans die each year due to medical errors, which certainly grabbed the attention of the media. A more contemporary analysis by the noted physician Danielle Ofri, MD, PhD, author of *When We Do Harm: A Doctor Confronts Medical Error,* indicated that the IOM account was grossly exaggerated, although she conceded that much work needs to be done to prevent medical errors. Scapegoating doctors and torturing them with malpractice suits is not in anyone's best interest.

For obvious reasons, then, spring engenders a range of emotions in me, often extreme. In one moment, I am recalling with delight the annual spring feeding of the koi. For no rhyme or reason, dark clouds roll in regarding the "jumper," and remorse sets in. Then memories of my father follow – mostly positive, but some negative. Thank goodness for the uplifting "Field of Dreams."

John Fox, in *Poetic Medicine,* affirms the therapeutic benefits of writing about difficult personal problems and struggles. He states: "Whatever form of therapy fits your particular temperament, externalizing your experience by creatively expressing it on paper, and if possible sharing it with someone special who listens well, is a way to state how things are, release old hurts, set healthy directions and develop potentials that make destructive past behavior or experience more a thing of the past."

The second chapter of *Poetic Medicine* is titled "The Same River Twice." It's a reference to Heraclitus, a Greek philosopher born in 544 BC, who said: "No man ever steps in the same river twice, for it's not the same river and he's not the same man." Every day, people change because they have new experiences that shape them. They encounter new people who influence them. People (like me) read books, take courses, and travel to new places – all of which change them and encourage them to open up and be more comfortable in their own skin. You cannot step into the same river twice, because both the individual and the river are constantly changing and interfacing in different ways.

They say spring showers bring May flowers. I'm glad when fall and football season have arrived.

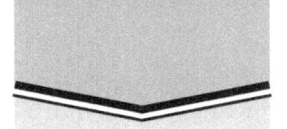

28

Cancel Me

Cancel me
Go ahead
Cancel me

Academics despise my remarks
Misinterpreted just like Karl Marx

Call me Republican, call me Democrat
Register me a scientific zealot

My intention was to start a debate
What resulted were claims of hate

My comments (out of context) appeared to condemn
Apparently, I've lost the right to say them

You've won the satisfaction
Of demanding a retraction (lest I face sanction)

Certainly, you've seen my flaws
Am I not allowed to have a cause?

My ideas were rather novel
Perhaps they caused you to unravel?

Experts can (and do) disagree in good faith
But your personal attacks are beginning to chafe

Cancel me
Go ahead
Cancel me

No doubt I have a different point of view
Who are you to say I have no clue?

Once I was a pioneer
Now my colleagues mock me, in unison they jeer

I've provided counsel for the defense
The facts you seek are not in evidence

Medicine has always been my dominion
I've been tried in the court of public opinion

I have the means to better human health
Why refuse my gesture of inestimable wealth?

First, do no harm
Second, sound the alarm

I've lived a noble doctor's life
What remains is sorrow and strife

My practice like a towering sculpture
Toppled by the cancel culture

29

Crying to be Heard:
Women in Emotional Pain

"Somebody's cryin' to be heard
And there's also someone who hears every word."
—Dave Mason (from "Cryin' to Be Heard," by Traffic)

Despite the intense suffering and horrific death and dying manifest in concentration camp victims, there is very little mention of crying in Viktor Frankl's psychological study of the Holocaust, *Man's Search for Meaning* (see essay 12). Any display of emotion was considered beyond the pale, yet there is probably no singular affect stronger, more moving, and more powerful than crying.

Near the end of Frankl's memoir, he reminds us that prisoners shed few tears in the camp, When the topic of crying is discussed, Frankl writes that tears bear witness to person's courage to suffer. However, only a few men in the camp realized that fact. Frankl recounts a powerful story about one prisoner who had wept: "The comrade … answered my question of how he had gotten over his edema [swelling] by confessing, 'I have wept it out of me.'"

Crying was verboten in concentration camps. Frankl was told that the only way to try and stay alive was to "look fit." But crying is a natural human response to adversity and other emotions – emotions that surely every prisoner experienced: sadness, pain, despair, and frustration. Nowhere was this more evident than at the Auschwitz concentration camp, where most children were gassed upon arrival. For those selected for labor, their mothers shouted, cried and banged heads against the wall as their children were transported to an unknown destination, according to Janina Kościuszkowa, a prisoner-doctor and witness to events. If anything, crying, outbursts, and other forms of emotional display were a sure way to call attention to prisoners and hasten their death.

Turning to the field of medicine, and by no means comparing it to events that transpired at Auschwitz or any other camp, I am struck by how often crying is overlooked — often deliberately — despite its therapeutic value and need for recognition. Crying can play a significant role in healing and achieving well-being. Research has shown that crying serves as an emotional release, provides pain relief, reduces stress, improves mood, and enhances communication. Encouraging a culture of acceptance and understanding around crying in medical settings can contribute to holistic and empathetic patient care.

Women are more prone than men to cry, and this does a disservice for women in distress. Crying women are often labeled "hysterical" or "emotional." Their complaints are taken less seriously. Their concerns are given short-shrift. Just when they may need more time with a caregiver to help process their fears, they are afforded less time, either because the caregiver is unsure how to react to a crying woman, and so retreats, or because they view it as someone else's job to console a woman in tears. Male physicians are particularly guilty on both counts, reacting more on bias than bedside manner.

British humanities and women's rights scholar Elinor Cleghorn argues in her book *Unwell Women* that the medical profession is mired in myth and misbeliefs about women. The history of medicine shows that men donning white coats have controlled the fate of women, and doctors' knowledge about women's' susceptibility to illness and disease has been shaped and distorted by prejudicial beliefs dating back to ancient Greece. Centuries ago, it was believed that a disconnected and "wandering womb" (uterus) was to blame for a variety of ailments, including excessive emotion, or hysteria. Hence, hysterectomy, from the Greek word "hysterika," meaning uterus, became a viable cure for physical and mental disorders in women.

My wife and I have experienced first-hand just how callous and unsympathetic some physicians can be, based on two incidents surrounding her pregnancies. The first incident occurred in 1986. My wife was in her first trimester, finally pregnant after suffering several miscarriages. She was seeing a fertility specialist, and he suggested we come into the office to confirm the pregnancy by ultrasound. The ultrasound technician turned to me and asked, "Would you be upset if I told you I think I see two heartbeats?" Miracle of miracles! Twins!

My wife was elated and she began to cry – happy tears. We returned to the waiting room, waiting to see the doctor. Tears continued to flow down my wife's cheeks, and I hugged her tight. No one in the waiting room inquired what was happening. None of the staff came from their station to check on us. No one offered my wife a box of Kleenex. No one – anyone – asked if everything was alright. They all assumed my wife had miscarried. After all, this was a fertility practice, where women were expected to have higher rates of miscarriages than in a typical OB-GYN office.

After what seemed like an eternity, my wife blurted out: "We're having twins!" A crowd of people came over to congratulate us, sharing in the joyous occasion. It was only then that kindness and good wishes were bestowed upon us. But had it been the misfortune of a miscarriage, or had the tears been the result of an unsuccessful attempt at becoming pregnant, there would have been no compassion.

Several years later, we suffered an agonizing loss: fetal demise. Everything was going fine until the OB-GYN informed my wife during a routine office visit that, at 20 weeks gestation, a heartbeat could not be heard. Later that night labor was induced to deliver the baby, a dead baby boy whom we had already named. The doctor let us view him briefly, and then they – the doctor and our baby – vanished. The nurses unemotionally looked after my wife while she and I wept. They handed us the discharge instructions and barely said "goodbye."

I've heard accounts from other women about how dispassionately their doctors treated them during labor and afterwards. My colleague's wife, a psychologist, nearly bled to death after a complicated delivery. She was left alone with unimaginable thoughts, her body ravaged and her spirit wounded. She was ignored throughout her entire episode of care, and she became psychologically traumatized. She and her (then) husband (my colleague), also a psychologist, decided to write a textbook: *Managing the Psychological Impact of Medical Trauma*. The book is the first to conceptualize medical trauma and provide healthcare practitioners with best practices for treating trauma in health care settings, trauma ranging from neglect to near-death experiences.

I commend my colleagues for producing such a textbook and lament that it had to be written in the first place. Why has it taken countless accounts from women in grief to finally validate their stories and call attention to the need for trauma-informed, patient-centered, care? How is it that some medical professionals cannot identify or deal with patients who cry and suffer and are at risk for PTSD and other mental health disorders following traumatic experiences – experiences that arise so easily and occur so often? Worse yet, why, when I researched the topic of medical trauma by doing a Google search, was the first hit an article in the *British Medical Journal* titled "Should Doctors Cry at Work?" Give me a break!

Crying holds a significant therapeutic value in medicine. Crying is a natural response to many feelings created by the hardships and uncertainty associated with physical and mental illnesses. Crying can be incorporated into comprehensive patient care plans and inform treatment. But women should not have to cry a river of tears to be accurately diagnosed, tended to with empathy, recognized for courage, and treated respectfully.

30

Reparations are Long Overdue in Medicine

Remediate wrongs and injustices to racial and ethnic minorities.

The *Philadelphia Inquirer* has been covering health inequities and potential remedial solutions for years. One recent story described how a new policy requires that patients' kidney function be estimated without taking their race into account, highlighting the case of a Black woman whose kidney transplant was delayed five years because the medical center relied on an outdated race-based formula to determine her kidney function, making the woman seem healthier than she really was (refer to essay 20).

In fact, hospitals nationwide have notified more than 3,700 Black people with kidney disease awaiting transplants of the error caused by an unnecessary modifier in calculating their estimated glomerular filtration rate (eGFR). By the end of this year, hospitals must go through their lists and recalculate the kidney function of all Black patients using a race-neutral formula. Transplant programs must review their lists of waitlisted candidates and credit those who may have been impacted by the use of the race-based calculation.

Other articles in the *Philadelphia Inquirer* have covered the failure of the Mütter Museum to repatriate the remains of Native Americans to their tribal descendants, as required by the Native American Graves Protection and Repatriation Act of 1990 (see essay 26). The world-famous Mütter museum in Philadelphia, Pennsylvania, houses many rare and one-of-a-kind medical artifacts and anomalies ostensibly used for educational purposes. But the museum has recently been caught in the crosshairs of the Act and uncertainty surrounding best practices for the ethical and respectful display of human remains. The remains of 49 (86%) of 57 Native Americans housed by the Mütter museum have not yet been made available for return to tribes, according to ProPublica's repatriation database as of October 2023.

The idea of remediating wrongs and injustices to racial and ethnic minorities, including indigenous peoples, dates back to the bible. Deuteronomy 15:12-15 states: "And when you release [Hebrew slaves], do not send them away empty-handed. Supply them liberally from your flock, your threshing floor, and your winepress."

In John Locke's *Second Treatise of Government* (1689), he wrote, "… he who hath received any damage has, besides the right of punishment common to him with other men, a particular right to seek reparation …"

Ta-Nehisi Coates made a compelling case for reparation in his 2014 award-winning essay "The Case for Reparations," published in *The Atlantic*. Coates wrote: "Two hundred fifty years of slavery. Ninety years of Jim Crow. Sixty years of separate but equal. Thirty-five years of racist housing policy. America will never be whole until we reckon with our compounding moral debts."

Jesse McCarthy, another powerful Black writer and critic on race and culture, authored *Who Will Pay Reparations on My Soul*, borrowing the title from Gil Scott-Heron's classic rap/song of the same title, which appeared on his 1970 debut album "A New Black Poet – Small Talk at 125th and Lenox." McCarthy, a Harvard professor, addresses the question of reparations by arguing that true progress will not come until Americans remake their institutions in the service of true equality.

Scott-Heron's version of reparations, however, clearly focuses on Native Americans, more than 50,000 of whom were dislocated from southeastern U.S. states to present-day Oklahoma, many dying along the Trail of Tears and while crossing the Mississippi River between 1830 and 1850 in forced compliance with the Indian Removal Act (see next essay).

> *"What about the red man*
> *Who met you at the coast?*
> *You never dig sharing;*
> *Always had to have the most.*
> *And what about Mississippi,*
> *The boundary of old?*
> *Tell me,*
> *Who'll pay reparations on my soul?"*

Scott-Heron's song remains as relevant, angry, and unanswered as ever – as we head into an election campaign where race, gender, and voting inequities – among many other inequalities – take center stage. And, oh yes, let's not forget health disparities.

Medical reparations are long overdue for Blacks, Latinos, Native Americans, Native Hawaiians, Native Alaskans, the LGBTQ+ community, and many other marginalized groups who have been targets of bias and discrimination by the medical profession. In my specialty of psychiatry alone, racial and ethnic bias in diagnosis is a huge problem affecting clinical decision-making and treatment planning.

Making reparations goes far beyond calling out one specialty, however. The impact of racism and bias found within health care as a whole, in terms of differential morbidity and mortality, is more than enough to justify reparations for injuries and psychological harm inflicted upon patients. Historical examples include not only biased diagnoses and algorithms flawed by "adjustments" for race but also the widespread misuse of biological concepts of race in research and education.

From cardiology to nephrology to obstetrics to urology, race has been used in algorithms to determine organ function, although there are often no racial or ethnic differences that inherently exist. Race correction actually reinforces long-established patient hierarchies in medicine. As the Inquirer article points out, correcting for race in the assessment of kidney function masks the complexity of the lived experience of societal neglect that damages health. The reality is that medicine and its technological foundations have been deeply intertwined with the histories and legacies of slavery, segregation, class oppression, and indigenous genocide.

Although reparations typically refer to financial compensation, reparative processes can also be embedded in policies directly or indirectly related to payments – for example, expanding Medicaid coverage, increasing reimbursement for diseases more prevalent in minority populations, funding community-driven interventions to address social determinants of health, and mandating community leaders on hospital governance boards and medical school admission committees. Equally important is the project of making medicine a more antiracist field.

Toni Martin, MD, an African American primary care physician with a multiethnic practice, was largely responsible for highlighting the fatal flaw behind the "adjustment factor" previously used to inflate kidney function (eGFR) in African Americans. She wrote "that even her patients became suspicious of the methodology, "born of years of experience with separate and unequal."

For example, Martin said, "Many of my patients and I are old enough to remember the days when our dense bones were proposed as the reason so few of us learned to swim. And yes, our bones, on average, are denser. But we couldn't swim, not because of our dense bones, but because the pools were segregated."

Martin further noted, "Some characteristics may be slightly different from race to race, on average, but generally, the average differences between two racial groups are smaller than the differences within a group." She implored the National Kidney Foundation to interpret all laboratory tests in a clinical context irrespective of race and reminded her colleagues "that the clinical context is always more important than a single number."

"That's our job as physicians," Martin concluded. In other words, to continue to push to remove racial bias from medical practice while paying reparations to our patients' souls.

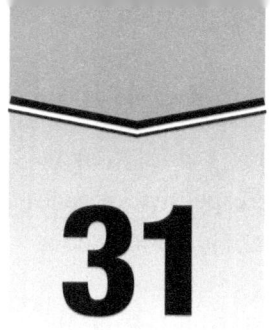

31

On Juneteenth I learned the Ugly Truth of My New Hometown. It Restored My Faith in Humanity.

We can't change history, but we can certainly improve upon it.

Most of the racially debated issues these days can be summed up by the terms "critical race theory" and "wokeism" – terms that have become the defining issues of our time even though half the people can't explain them and the other half use them for political gain to dictate how history is taught, stripping it of any mention of slavery, racism, and LGBTQ+ people. So, I'd like to reframe the debate and ask whether there is a middle ground where we can reject racist hatred while attempting to understand it and teach the truth about past social injustices to present and future generations – to keep our children from hating our country and each other.

I thought this was a noble proposition given that my wife and I recently moved to a southern town and attended its celebration of Juneteenth (2023), which brought the community together with arts, dance, music, spoken word and an educational panel discussion. I learned that our town, officially known as Indian Trail, takes its name from the city's history as a trade route that connected Petersburg, Virginia, to the Waxhaw Indian settlement and nearby gold mining areas in North Carolina near Charlotte.

There is also some debate whether Indian Trail is situated along the path referred to as the "Trail of Tears," a network of routes used for the forced displacement of approximately 60,000 Native Americans from the southeast U.S. to present-day Oklahoma between 1830 and 1850. It didn't strike me as a coincidence that my hometown would be named "Indian Trail" unless it was somehow part of the actual "Trail of Tears."

One of the likely routes comprising the "Trail of Tears" bisects Indian Trail and is now a major thoroughfare named "Independence Boulevard" – an incredible slight to the Cherokee Nation – over 5,000 of whom perished during their westward journey across the Mississippi River, many originating from North Carolina and buried in unmarked graves along the way. Even worse, Independence Boulevard is officially named Andrew Jackson Highway in homage to the seventh president of the U.S. who signed the Indian Removal Act into law and was a prominent slave trader considered by many to be an "ideal slave-owner."

Driving west on the "Highway" takes me to uptown Charlotte in about 20 minutes. In the same amount of time, heading east, I can reach historic Monroe, North Carolina, a city marked by violence against the minority Black community during the civil rights movement years of the 1960s and where people still defend the display of the Confederate flag and monuments.

As I learned about the dark history surrounding my newly adopted hometown I thought, "Who will make reparations for the Native Americans and African Americans so unfairly treated here over the past two centuries?" Although I have long known about injustices embedded in the fabric of our society, it was Juneteenth that crystalized the connection between racism and the medical profession – by heightening my awareness of the case for reparations in general, and the case for health reparations, in particular

While Juneteenth is widely observed as a celebration of Black American history and heritage, commemorating the emancipation of the last of enslaved African Americans on June 19, 1865, the holiday also highlights health impacts of structural racism – namely, the disparity in health care and health literacy access that continues to contribute to chronic disease, hospitalization and mortality among Black Americans. The toll that health inequity has taken on the African American community is extensive, as reflected in data compiled by the Centers for Disease Control and Prevention.

Additional data presented by The Commonwealth Fund showed a surge in preventable deaths in every state in 2021, fueled mainly by COVID-19, with Black, Hispanic, and American Indian/Alaska Native people experiencing the highest mortality rates in many places. Researchers also noted that many Americans with mental health needs face barriers to obtaining care, and millions of people – particularly in the South – are wallowing in medical debt.

I was saddened to learn that North Carolina does not have the best track record when it comes to healthy living: the state ranks 39th in the country for access to mental health treatment, and it ranks in the lower half of all states in overall health outcomes and healthy behaviors.

Our town's celebration of Juneteenth reminded me that health inequalities also extend to the LGBTQ+ community. Many LGBTQ+ individuals continue to face stigma and discrimination based on their sexual orientation, gender identity, or gender expression. As a result, research shows that the LGBTQ+ population struggles disproportionately with mental illness, substance use, and suicide.

Medical bias and social stigma particularly towards transgender and gender diverse (TGD) people is widely prevalent in the U.S. The TGD community is faced with health disparities, discrimination, harassment, and lack of access to quality health care. Gender-affirming care should be regarded as health care that can reduce health disparities and save lives. This cannot be understated in light of the increasing violence against the LGBTQ+ community and LGBTQ+ people of color – particularly transgender people – who are disproportionately affected by hate crimes.

Individuals and organizations that attempt to limit access to treatment or ban therapy intended to maintain the health and welfare of marginalized groups – African Americans, Native Americans, Latinx, Native Hawaiians, Native Alaskans, LGBTQ+ and TGD – restrict their lives and freedoms. These groups must be stopped, along with their hate-fueled ideologies, until they learn to embrace the incredible diversity and heterogeneity of the U.S. population. To me, that is the essence of Juneteenth: a time to reflect on past racial injustices and rectify ongoing health inequities in wide swaths of the populace – and maybe, just maybe, help restore our faith in humanity.

32

Medicine on Fire

My heart's on fire
For my patients
For all who were in my presence
Anxious and depressed
Suffering in pain
Wanting healing
Receiving none
Reminding them
"The absence of evidence
Is not evidence of absence."

The heart of the matter
Could be about forgiveness
But also
Decency and respect
Compassion and caring
Wanting attention
Receiving none
Pleading
"Treat me
And not the chart."

Medicine on fire
Burns less brightly
Embers dying
Crackling
Cold
Wanting kindling
Receiving none
Flames extinguished
"What is to give light."
must endure burning."*

*End-quote by Viktor Frankl

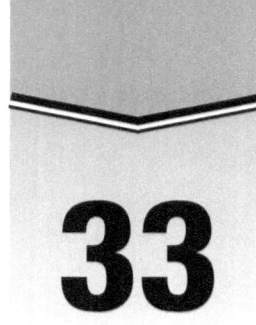

33

The Essence of Health Narratives, Including Poetry, from the Patient's Perspective

If you write, they will read.

In the vast universe of all that has been written, writing about loss, illness, and death is probably second only to writing about intimacy, relationships, and longing. In the world of narrative medicine, the order is reversed. Patients are harnessing the power of writing, sharing, and telling stories of health and sickness using personal narratives to navigate illness, trauma, and grief. The experience of being ill is made less isolating by connecting with like-minded individuals and communities moving through life transitions and illness, those who provide sustenance on this difficult journey.

Health narratives, also known as illness narratives or medical narratives, are not merely stories patients tell about their experiences with illness, medical conditions, or health care-related events. These narratives also include a patient's understanding and interpretation of their illness, the challenges they face, their coping strategies, and their overall experience with and passage through the health care system.

The essence of health narratives lies in their potential to provide a holistic view of a patient's health, beyond just the clinical aspects. They encompass the emotional, psychological, social, and cultural dimensions of health, thus offering a more comprehensive understanding of a patient's overall well-being.

In my experience, patients and physicians write narratives for similar reasons, especially if physicians have experienced the health system from both sides, i.e., as provider *and* patient. Here is a brief accounting of why patients write medical narratives:

1. **Enhancing patient-provider communication.** Health narratives can facilitate better communication between patients and health care providers by providing a platform for patients to express their experiences, concerns, and expectations. This can help practitioners to understand the patient's perspective and provide more personalized care.

2. **Patient empowerment.** By sharing their stories, patients can feel a sense of control and empowerment in their health care journey. It can also encourage self-reflection and self-awareness, which can be beneficial for self-management of chronic conditions.

3. **Education and awareness.** Health narratives can serve as educational tools, providing insights into the lived experiences of individuals with specific health conditions. This can increase awareness and understanding among health care professionals, patients, and the general public.

4. **Research and policy development.** Researchers and policymakers can use health narratives to gain insights into the patient experience, which can inform the development of patient-centered care models, health policies, and health promotion strategies.

5. **Therapeutic benefits.** The process of recounting one's health journey can have enormous therapeutic benefits, such as emotional catharsis and reduced stress. It can also help patients make sense of their experiences and find meaning in their illness. Studies actually show that patients who read

poetry together experience decreased pain and symptoms of depression. Even if patients choose not to write about their health, or if sickness prevents them from writing, reading poetry may plant seeds for their writing when the time is ripe.

A few words about poems are in order. We can debate until the cows come home whether poetry should be considered a form of narrative. Technically, it isn't. There are three major types of creative writing (essay 5): fiction, creative nonfiction, and poetry. Each has its place in the literary annals, and students applying to graduate fine arts (MFA) schools are usually asked to choose a particular medium for specialized concentration. Narrative medicine is considered a subset of creative nonfiction. However, the genre borrows many of its tools from poetry – for example, the use of simile, metaphor, imagery, word choice and emotional expression – and poems are firmly rooted in the field of narrative medicine.

There is no doubt in my mind that patients write more poems than physicians, although I do not know any statistic or research that can back me up. But that's not the point. The point is that physicians should understand that if they encourage their patients to write about their illnesses – and they should encourage them to write – including sharing in their patients' works, patients are likely to bring them poetry as well as narratives, and physicians should be somewhat knowledgeable about poetry and delight in reading their patients' poems and give feedback.

Certified poetry therapist John Fox suggests that "poem-making can be a way to remember we are flesh and blood." Writing poems is a way to tap into our vulnerability when we are seriously ill, a vulnerability generally disregarded by modern health care systems preoccupied with technology. Fox criticizes – rightly so – any "medical system that displaces human contact and sense of community with an intense reliance on machines and drugs." Writing poems under those conditions may allow patients to begin to live creatively rather than think about it, he observes.

I like the poem Fox chooses to introduce the third chapter of his book *Poetic Medicine*. The chapter is titled "Poetic Tools for Your Healing Journey," and the poem is "The Remedies," by Native American Joseph Bruchac. The opening and closing verses are as follows:

> *Half on the Earth, half in the heart,*
> *the remedies for all the things*
> *which grieve us wait for those who know*
> *the words to use to find them.*

> * * * *

> *Half on the Earth, half in the heart,*
> *the remedies for all our pains*
> *wait for the songs of healing.*

Words are as important as medicine in the healing process. Physicians should never forget it.

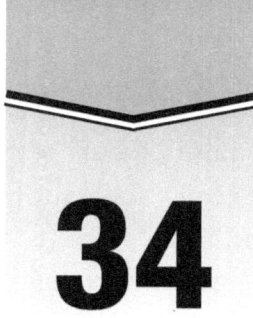

34

Expressive Writing Reduces Caregiver Stress

Write. It's doctor's orders!

Today, more than one in five Americans are caregivers, providing care to an adult or child with special needs at some time in the past 12 months. Given this sobering statistic, I'm surprised we do not see as many health narratives written by caregivers as, say, doctors and patients, at least not in print.

Caregiving is emotionally draining. However, writing when you are in a caregiving role is one of handful ways to console and take care of yourself, to improve your well-being. Whether you are a caregiver in a hospital or home or places in-between, writing can be a form of nurturing and renewal, an answer to the question that so many caregivers ask: "Who will take care of me?" Let's face it, caregiving can make your own health worse, so say about a quarter of the people in caregiving roles.

Once every five years, AARP takes the pulse of caregivers in the United States. The most recent survey is from 2020. Although the results may be tinged by COVID-19, the flavor comes through. Here are the main takeaways as discussed in the executive summary:

- Nearly one in five (19%) of Americans are providing unpaid care to an adult with health or functional needs.

- More Americans (24%) are caring for more than one person, up from 18% in 2015.
- More family caregivers (26%) have difficulty coordinating care, up from 19% in 2015.
- More Americans (26%) are caring for someone with Alzheimer's disease or dementia, up from 22% in 2015.
- More Americans (23%) say caregiving has made their own health worse, up from 17% in 2015.
- Family caregiving spans across all generations, including Boomers, Gen-X, Gen-Z, Millennials, and Silent.
- 61% of family caregivers are also working.

The AARP survey also paints a picture of the many different faces of caregivers stepping up to help family and friends: ethnic minorities, LGBTQ+, students, and so on – essentially individuals from all walks of life. Career disruption and "losses in living" are common consequences of caregiving. Unfortunately, caregiving is a growing reality in the U.S. as the proportion of older adults with cognitive impairments increases, and helping resources decrease, including eldercare and health insurance.

Caregivers report physical, emotional, and financial strain, with 2 in 10 reporting they feel alone. Thus, support for caregivers and their recipients is especially critical to counter the epidemic of loneliness. The AARP survey notes that: "Without greater explicit support for caregivers, their overall responsibilities will likely intensify and place greater pressures on individuals within families, especially as baby boomers move into old age." That's why, despite various solutions proposed to address this national crisis – many of them complex and politically non-starters – something as simple as writing about the caregiving experience and sharing those experiences with other caregivers can bear so much fruit.

There are very few national, centralized well-organized movements of writers or writing programs for caregivers, but there are certainly local chapters. Most of them are organized by communities, where all comers are welcome in person or online, or by disease type, e.g., Alzheimer's, childhood disabilities, and others. Some offer weekend retreats and workshops (who has the time for a "retreat," you ask?). One workshop advertises: "No rules. Just write. Write time. Write place. Write now." Here are some examples of caregivers who participated in that group writing program:

- A woman taking care of her mother who has Alzheimer's disease.
- A mother taking care of a child who has developmental delays.
- A husband whose wife sustained a brain injury in a car accident.
- A father whose son has a serious mental illness.
- A woman whose sister died from cancer and who, like her fellow caregivers, wants to begin sorting out those experiences in writing.

Research shows that family caregivers who list self-care as a priority can better provide care, are at lower risk of burning out and becoming ill, and find more joy in their role as a caregiver. Writing is a form of self-care; it creates a sacred space and nourishes and restores our vitality. While taking care of a loved one, you may have lost much of your former lifestyle including social supports and activities. There is a good chance you are feeling stressed and isolated and need to develop or acquire healthful self-care practices. Think of writing as care for the caregiver, a good nosh, or chicken soup for the soul.

An interesting observation about narratives of family caregiving is that diverse themes emerge, suggesting that caregivers interpret different meanings despite often similar experiences. In addition, a narrative approach may help caregivers transition into the role needed for coping with the eventual loss of a loved one. Although expressive writing cannot change the reality of a loss, it can help caregivers to reframe the significance or story related to that loss.

Even if you don't think of yourself as a writer, you have a story. A woman from British Columbia wrote:

"I started just writing stories about what was going on; my thoughts, my feelings. Some of those actually became published in the local senior's newspaper, which I'm grateful for. As it turned out, the published articles not only helped me, they helped others as well."

So, organize your thoughts on paper, and if you can do it in the company of others who "get it," so much the better.

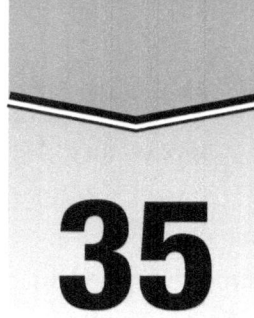

35

A Mother's Journey Advocating for Children with Chronic Lyme Disease

— by Cheryl R. Lazarus

My wife's struggle for the health of our children.

My husband, a physician, and I have four wonderful children – a son and three daughters. I look back over the past decade and wonder, "Why?" Why did my daughters contract Lyme disease and not my son or husband? Why was it so difficult to establish a diagnosis? Why are doctors specializing in treating patients with Lyme disease considered pariahs, while conventional doctors may not consider the diagnosis and often miss it? Why do insurance companies deny treatment for long-term Lyme disease? Why was it so difficult to get help from a profession that was supposed to help people?

I counsel and console other mothers going through similar situations – caring for children affected by Lyme disease and other chronic conditions – and they always ask how I managed to get through the ordeal. I managed because I am, and always will be, a mom. I did it for my children – they needed advocates when they couldn't do it themselves. I had no other option. If not, I don't know where my daughters would be today.

A wise woman once told me (when I felt at the end of my rope): "Don't waste your energy being upset by the people who don't 'get it.' They will never understand until those individuals experience something like you did." Unfortunately, I have found this to be true, but it shouldn't have to be this way. Doctors shouldn't have to literally walk in a patient's shoes to understand their despair, but many need to gain empathy and compassion, seemingly lost along the way.

If I could say one thing to the many doctors I have seen on my journey, it would be that they need to listen to their patients and their families. Don't brush them off and discount their opinions, believing that the only correct answer is the physician's. That "see a mental health professional" recommendation becomes indelibly stamped into the medical record and poisons the well. It biases future doctors and undermines patients' integrity and self-confidence, or what little remains of it.

Get to know your patients before you pass judgment. Check their charts first and find out what they have been through. Ask them about prior medical encounters and experiences. Before you write off a patient, realize that test results aren't always accurate and symptoms can be vexing; they don't always comport to a readily discernible disorder.

I had lost count of the doctors who hadn't checked my daughters' records before they entered the exam room. Once, one of my daughters saw a gastroenterologist. He told her, "You have irritable bowel syndrome." She calmly eyed him and said, "I don't have a bowel" (she had had a colectomy), to which his response was, "May I ask why not?" The physician never offered an apology or explanation for his terrible miscue.

A great doctor once explained that patients who suffer are the real experts. I have met so many doctors brimming with knowledge gleaned from textbooks and research studies, but they ignored the plight of their patients. Isn't it the ability to relate to patients' subjective experiences and consider their notion of what ails them, as well as their fears of the disease, that is part of the "art" of medicine? I would rather a doctor be honest and tell me they are unsure what is going on and make a referral than pretend to have all the answers. Instead of subjecting my family to the pain and anguish of unmet promises and false hopes, I would respect that.

To all those doctors who have listened and been there for us, I want to say "thank you." My daughters were so profoundly affected by Lyme disease and their exchanges with medical professionals – both positive and negative – that they decided to enter the medical profession. They are the bravest people I know; the doctors who listened to and helped them are our heroes!

36

How (and when) to Fire Your Doctor

Lessons learned the hard way.

Soon after beginning my psychiatric residency, I encountered a patient with all the hallmarks of borderline personality disorder: volatile relationships, emotional instability, and repeated threats of suicide. I asked my supervisor, "How do you treat these patients?" "Art," he replied, tongue-in-cheek, "you refer them!"

As a psychiatric resident, I did not have that luxury. I was required to take all comers. But I did remember his advice once I completed my residency and joined the faculty of my medical school alma mater. Now *I* was able to saddle residents with some of the most undesirable, if not vexing patients, in all of medicine.

It's sad to admit that there are several other ways doctors unload undesirable patients. One way is to screen them. They require the patient to submit all pertinent medical records and review the records, determining whether they want to accept the challenge – or not.

Another way is for doctors to advertise themselves as consultants. Consultants are not patients' doctors, at least not yet. Their purpose is to take a history and physical, arrive at a diagnosis, and relate treatment recommendations to the primary doctor. Afterward, a consultant may accept the patient into their practice if they are inclined.

Doctors who are the cream of the crop can close their practice to new patients. But they can always instruct front office personnel to tell new patients they may be able to "squeeze" them in, depending on the circumstances. Then they can revert to the consultant role and steer patients to a more "suitable" provider if they choose not to treat them.

Once a physician is confronted with an undesirable patient, they can always escape through the door – "step out the back, Jack" – saving face by claiming a lack of expertise. The following euphemisms have proven effective:

- "Your problems really don't coincide with my area of expertise. May I refer you to specialist?"
- "I would be doing you a disservice if I took your case. I really think you need to see someone with more experience."
- Your medical issues are complex and extensive. A concierge physician is your best bet."

Perhaps the most common way doctors jettison undesirable patients is to neglect or abandon them. Neglecting them is easy; they don't return their phone calls or emails. Abandoning patients, on the other hand, is more difficult and raises ethical issues. At the very least, dumping patients requires that doctors provide them with written notification of termination, a suitable list of alternative providers, and an offer to treat the patient in the event of an emergency until a replacement physician is found.

My daughter had a serious health problem, as I discuss in the following essay. Her doctor chose the path of neglect and abandonment. She lodged a formal complaint with the state medical licensing agency. I applauded her actions.

Perhaps the best course of action is to fire your doctor before they fire you. A patient fired me for neglecting my plants (essay 3). Scanning my office, she remarked, "If you can't take care of your plants, how do you expect to take care of me?"

Here are 10 signs it's time to fire your doctor:

1. The chemistry is not right. You don't feel you can relate to your physician. They relate better to the electronic medical record system that to you.
2. Your waiting time to see the doctor is consistently too long, or they give you too little face time.
3. You can't reach your doctor when you really need them. You're left hanging in an emergency, or told to dial "911," or worse yet, "988."
4. The doctor's treatment doesn't make sense to you. They become defensive or indignant when questioned.
5. They don't share specifics with you, e.g., results of lab tests and imaging studies.
6. Your complaints fall on deaf ears; your concerns are minimized, trivialized, or not addressed at all.
7. The office staff – the gatekeepers – are rude, patronizing, or condescending.
8. You question whether your doctor really knows you, because you keep covering the same ground.
9. Your preferences are not included in treatment planning.
10. Your doctor does not coordinate your care with other doctors.

In the cult classic, *The House of God*, the author, psychiatrist Samuel Shem (a pseudonym for Stephen Joseph Bergman, MD), recommends denying hospital admission to undesirable patients in the emergency room, or transferring them elsewhere. Several decades later, a humbled Dr. Shem reflects how he has learned the essence of medical care, and life: it is "connection." Shem encourages doctors to put themselves in their patients' shoes and speak up if they see something wrong in the healthcare system. They should remember the patient is never only the patient – the patient is the world, with family, friends, community, and history.

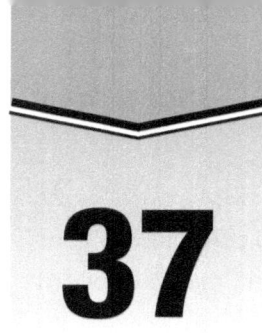

37

Abandoned – Not Once, But Twice – By the Same Practice

An unthinkable tale of woe.

Abandonment is often the path of least resistance for physicians who are confronted with undesirable patients, e.g., those who are disruptive or violent, non-adherent to therapy, or destitute and uninsured. Unfortunately, complex and challenging patients are often mistakenly lumped into this category. My daughter, Heather, is a case in point. She gave me permission to write about her experience.

Heather has a serious GI motility disorder. She has undergone surgery many times. Heather is a challenging patient, not only because of her medical condition, but also because she is a physician assistant and she has expert medical knowledge.

In June 2016, Heather experienced complications from previous abdominal surgery. She required corrective surgery, but her surgeon disagreed with the commonly recommended procedure. Shortly afterward, Heather received a letter from her surgeon. It read, in part, "I believe that the relationship between our practice and you has become significantly strained. In light of this, I regretfully feel I can no longer serve as your provider. Your insurance company is able to assist you with the selection of a medical provider of your choosing. I will, of course, be available for emergencies during this time of transition."

Heather was stunned that her surgeon dismissed her for his failure to perform the recommended surgery. She sought the help of a different surgeon, who performed the necessary procedure that Heather's surgeon was unwilling to do. She did well for 18 months, but another complication set in. Unfortunately, her new surgeon had become quite ill and was no longer practicing. There were a small number of colorectal surgeons in Heather's town, so she made an appointment with a surgeon in the practice that had previously terminated her, a surgeon that was new to her but practiced in the original group. In fact, the surgeon who had dismissed Heather from the practice was no longer affiliated with that group.

The new surgeon saw Heather on September 19 and 29, 2017, and he scheduled surgery on October 19, 2017. On October 2, 2017, Heather experienced symptoms typical of a partial abdominal obstruction – severe abdominal pain, nausea, and vomiting. She became frightened and called her surgeon, but Heather was only able to speak with the nurse practitioner. Heather and the nurse practitioner had a disagreement. Heather wanted to come to the emergency room (ER) to be evaluated in case she needed surgery earlier than planned. The nurse practitioner informed Heather that, even if she came to the ER, her surgeon would not be available to operate until October 19, as planned. Heather explained that it was not her intention to circumvent the scheduled surgery or move it up. Rather, she wanted relief from her pain and nausea, as well as a medical evaluation for a possible "acute abdomen."

Heather managed to weather the storm without going to the ER. Two days later, she called the office to give them an update, and she asked to speak to a nurse practitioner other than the one she had had the disagreement with. Heather also wanted to learn more about the "fast-track" (no narcotic) post-operative program the surgeon had planned for her. She was put on hold. The "disagreeable" nurse practitioner came on the line and told Heather that, because she had considered consulting a different surgeon in the ER, and because she had questioned the fast-track program, her surgery was being cancelled. The doctor never spoke to Heather, and he never responded to my phone calls and emails seeking an explanation for cancelling Heather's surgery.

Several days later, Heather received a letter terminating her from the practice – again! It was the same form letter she had received a year and a half ago, except this time, the surgeon did not offer to be available for emergencies (that paragraph was omitted from the letter). Fortunately, Heather was quickly seen by another surgeon, albeit several hundred miles away. The surgeon promptly scheduled the required operation, and she had a good outcome.

Clearly, Heather was abandoned by the practice, not once, but twice, according to standard legal definitions of abandonment, i.e., "the unilateral termination of a physician-patient relationship by the physician (or other healthcare provider) without proper notice to the patient when there is still the necessity of continuing attention." In a formal complaint to the state medical licensing agency, Heather wrote, "I may not be an expert, but I know this is not how patient-centered care was designed. Complex patients and patients perceived as challenging or difficult to treat should not be labeled 'non-compliant' or any other term and summarily dismissed from treatment, especially at their most medically vulnerable moment, when surgical intervention is required."

Heather never heard back from the medical board.

Strike three.

38

Seeking Closure in Psychotherapy

Learning to live with ambiguity.

I had known my analyst, whom I'll call Stewart (not his real name), since medical school. He was the professor I mentioned in the preface, the one who told our class "you all belong here." Stewart's receptive ear and stalwart guidance helped me sort out the intricacies of a non-clinical career in medicine. He helped me prepare for, and overcome my resistance to, relocating to another city for a significant job opportunity: I became the first-ever vice president of behavioral health at a large mid-western insurance company.

Before leaving town, my wife joined me in therapy. Stewart was a master at marital and family therapy, often practicing conjointly with his wife, Serena (not her real name), herself a clinical counselor with a master's degree in social work.

I had an argument with my wife about one of my passions – an obsession according to her – my ever-growing collection of music on CDs. My wife felt that several thousand CDs provided sufficient listening pleasure for a lifetime, yet I was inclined to expand my collection. Stewart always strove for compromise between couples, but this time he was unable to help us strike an accord. An avid devotee of literature and the humanities, Stewart confessed he was struggling with his own obsession – collecting books!

My therapeutic relationship with Stewart ostensibly ended around the turn of the century, when I departed for my new job in the midwest. Before I left, I shaved my beard of nearly 20 years. I had always considered my beard a symbol of our bond. My facial hair marked a lasting identification with Stewart. He had a beard the entire time I had known him. I started growing mine soon after I began therapy with him, while still a psychiatry resident. However, I read an article purporting that physicians working in corporations were better off without a beard, because a beard could create mistrust in non-physician executives. So, I shaved my beard, and I have remained clean-shaven to this day.

I kept in touch with Stewart over the years, after therapy was terminated. We communicated through old-fashioned letter writing, and sometimes Stewart would send me notes written on his R_x pad. Stewart revealed more of himself through our correspondence. We kept each other appraised of our growing families and activities. Stewart was a sports enthusiast who played tennis well into his 80's. He and Serena traveled extensively. Hawaii was their favorite vacation spot. My son and his family live in Honolulu. Go figure!

I frequently shared my articles with Stewart, usually those about medical leadership and opportunities for physicians interested in medical management. In 2014, he wrote: "Art, you should be proud of yourself and your career – you've done well. Good I could help. Of course, I read all of your articles and enjoy them immensely. You're direct and to the point. Your recent article on PTSD in physicians [discussed in essay 24] is excellent and needs to be read by all M.D.'s and caretakers." It's no small measure that Stewart's encouragement factored into my writing as an extracurricular activity.

Stewart received numerous accolades for teaching, including the Lindback Award for Distinguished Teaching. In 2013, he was honored for nearly 60 years of psychiatry service. He retired in 2015, and after his death in 2018, I made a contribution to one of his designated charities. I could not attend the Celebration of His Life because it coincided with my youngest daughter's wedding. However, Serena sent me a beautiful thank you note. It read, in part, "Art, I saw your [online] comments in the funeral house guestbook. Stewart admired you, your work and your work ethic. You were special."

Serena's use of the word "special" was uncanny. Did she know that I needed Stewart to view me as "special," that it was a critical part of the transference underlying my therapeutic work? Did Stewart ever tell Serena that I longingly wanted him to think of me as "special." Did they talk about me in their home, apart from therapy, perhaps at the dinner table?

I will never know, and fortunately Stewart helped me live with uncertainty so that after he passed, I was able to resist the temptation to ask Serena whether Stewart had ever mentioned the issue of my "specialness." Stewart helped me discover an inner resilience to handle life's unknowns and inevitable twists and turns. If one defines closure as an individual's desire for ironclad knowledge and an absence of ambiguity in life, then Stewart's legacy is that finding "closure" is at best elusive, and I'm okay with that ending.

It's believed that most worthwhile destinations start with an amazing journey. Psychotherapy is no exception, as long as the tour guide knows the terrain. Stewart was an exceptional tour guide. He embodied all the characteristics considered prerequisite for a therapist: kindness, compassion, understanding, and critical reasoning. His therapeutic skills saved lives and marriages. He was truly an unsung hero, forever worthy to "serve the suffering" – the motto of the Alpha Omega Alpha Honor Medical Society, to which we both belonged.

I was fortunate to glimpse Stewart's personal and family life, a rarity for patients in therapy, especially those in analysis. I had many interactions with Stewart outside of therapy, mainly through social functions held by the psychiatry department during my residency and afterward. Stewart was an expert at maintaining therapeutic boundaries despite wearing many different professional hats.

Stewart and Serena's mutual love and support spanned a marriage of 67 years. Their son was my medical school classmate. He practices psychiatry in California. Stewart and Serena's daughter and grandson are also physicians. Two medical school classes including mine dedicated their yearbooks to Stewart. My yearbook concludes: "He taught us to be human, to face the inequities and suffering encountered in medicine, while preserving some perspective, while maintaining a sense of humor. [He] has taught us to smile."

Stewart was special. Me, I'm just ordinary.

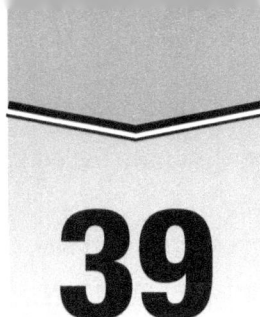

Rock and Roll as a Form of Narrative Healing

"It's only rock 'n' roll but I like it."
—Keith Richards/Mick Jagger

Paul Simon sings about feeling "crapped out" at four in the morning as he begins to write a song. Here I am, before sunrise, beginning to write an essay on the significance of rock and roll music to illness narratives, specifically, the way in which singer-songwriters have captured elements of illness in their music.

I am sticking to rock and roll music because that's the genre I know best, but certainly country, folk and especially blues music would also be appropriate categories. Quoting blues legend Willie Dixon: "The blues are the roots and the other musics are the fruits." And although jazz is mostly free of lyrics, a 2022 tribute album to the late jazz pianist Carla Bley is titled "Healing Power" in recognition of the powerful effects of jazz music on the mind and body and the fact that aficionados often turn to jazz for its invigorating feeling.

I am writing about rock and roll music because I grew up during the "British Invasion," and I entered my teen years during the "Summer of Love." I am also breaking a long-standing, self-imposed writing rule, which is to write what I know about rather than write what I want to know about. I'm may not be an expert in rock and roll music, but the "liner notes" in my hundreds of LPs and thousands of CDs have fueled my knowledge.

Before I discuss a few choice songs, I will review how rock and roll music and song lyrics can be viewed as a form of narrative medicine. Consider the following six dimensions relative to the narrative that can be captured in rock and roll music:

1. **Expression of Emotion**: Rock and roll songs often express deep emotions and personal experiences, including those related to health and illness. These songs can help patients articulate their feelings about their medical conditions, which can be therapeutic and promote healing.

2. **Artistic Expression**: Rock musicians often create music with a flair, and this appeals to patients. Musicians have been said to possess an "artistic temperament." Before many became famous, they studied in schools of theatre and design (The Talking Heads). Some musicians were English literature (Steely Dan) or film majors (Jim Morrison) in college.

3. **Connection and Empathy**: Listening to rock and roll songs about health and illness can help physicians and other healthcare providers better understand and empathize with the experiences of their patients. This can improve patient-provider communication and enhance the quality of care. Some physicians do procedures with rock music in the background to help them focus and concentrate or relive stress during an operation.

4. **Patient Identity and Experience**: Rock and roll song lyrics can provide insights into the identity and experiences of patients, including their hopes, fears, and coping mechanisms. This can help healthcare providers tailor their treatment approaches to meet the unique needs of each patient. Erik Eriksson may as well have had rock musicians in mind when he coined the term

"identity crisis," because rock stars suffer emotionally as much if not more than their listeners.

5. **Education and Awareness**: Rock and roll songs can raise awareness about specific health issues and promote health education. They can also challenge societal perceptions and stigmas related to certain diseases. Nowhere is this more evident than in the direct-to-consumer television commercials using rock songs to promote new medications for illness once considered taboo, e.g., HIV/AIDS.

6. **Community and Support**: Rock and roll songs about health and illness can foster a sense of community among patients, providing them with emotional support and reducing feelings of isolation. Just as Taylor Swift has her "Swifties," so, too, in my day did the Grateful Dead have "Dead Heads." They felt less "bad" going down the road, "where the climate suits [their] clothes [and] the water tastes like wine."

Some of my favorite rock songs have deep roots in health and illness narratives. I hope you listen to them at your leisure, assuming you are not already familiar with them, and explore other types of music that are the "fruits" of the tree.

"The Bottle" – This is Gil Scott-Heron's great song about the afflictions of alcohol use disorder. It is one of the finest disease awareness songs ever written. Scott-Heron's "Home is Where the Hatred Is" is an equally poignant piece about heroin addiction. Scott-Heron was bedeviled by his own addiction problems for many years. He died in 2011 from complications of HIV illness. Scott-Heron was an author, poet and musicologist. His music incorporated elements of rock, jazz and soul, and he was dubbed the "Godfather of Rap" for creating the genre.

"T.B. Sheets" – Before the extended musical odyssey of "Astral Weeks," 22-year-old-old Van Morrison chronicled this extended jam-laden narrative (it is nearly 10-minutes long) about a visit to the room of a young woman, Julie, dying of tuberculosis. While not exactly sad in tone, its repetition grows more harrowing with every bar and beat. This is a blues-infused rock song drenched in death – the bed sheets reek of tuberculosis ("T.B.") – and a soundtrack hallmark of Martin Scorsese's 1999 film, *Bringing Out the Dead*. Legend has it that Morrison himself broke down in tears after first recording it.

"She's Lost Control" – Ian Curtis was the troubled genius and front man of the post-punk British band Joy Division, which made only two studio albums: "Unknown Pleasures" and "Closer." "She's Lost Control" is a song from the first album. It is about a young woman living with the chaos of a seizure disorder and the fear of seizures. Curtis knew the young woman through his work at a rehabilitation center. His awareness and experiences of the stigma endured by individuals suffering from neurological impairments formed the lyrical inspiration for the song. "She's Lost Control" also carries no small amount of authenticity given that Curtis himself suffered from epilepsy, including seizures that manifested on stage. Curtis' seizure disorder contributed to his suicide death in 1980 at the age of 23, along with marital problems and depression.

"Lyme Life" – Lyme disease is caused by a bite from a tick infected with the Lyme bacteria. The tick is commonly known as a "deer tick" because it parasitizes the white-tailed deer. If the infection is not diagnosed and treated early, within the first several weeks, it can become chronic and more difficult to treat. Symptom flares of fatigue, pain, sweats, palpitations and mild cognitive problems can keep individuals from functioning at their full capacity. This was the case with a half-dozen musicians who have struggled openly with Lyme disease, most notably Daryl Hall (Hall & Oates) and Jesse Colin

Young (The Youngbloods), the latter writing "Lyme Life" in 2015 and recording it on his 2019 album "Dreamers." In a Healthline interview, Hall referred to the management of Lyme disease as a "scandal" due to the fact that some doctors refuse to acknowledge the chronic form of the illness.

"The Real Me" – The inability to receive effective treatment doesn't need to be the subject of every song about doctors, although it often is. Consider "The Real Me" from The Who, in which the lyrics describe the thoughts of a frustrated "mod" who exclaims: "Can you see the real me, doctor?" – a youthful cry for understanding and validation. The sentiment reflects a feeling many patients have in treatment or in therapy. Pete Townshend, the song's composer, has described it as an autobiographical song, with the lyrics reflecting his own search for authenticity and the challenges he faced in finding his true self.

I initially became enamored with rock and roll music for the catchy melodies and the craze surrounding "Bealtemania." The lyrics were secondary because I wasn't old enough to appreciate their meaning and the music tended to drown them out. It was later in my life, definitely by the time I was practicing medicine, that I began to pay closer attention to rock and roll lyrics and came to realize how they are a testament to the power of music and storytelling in healing.

Scroll the online comments of viewers of YouTube videos of the aforementioned artists and songs as well as other illness-related songs to gain a sense of their impact. Upon watching a live performance of Curtis performing "She's Lost Control," a mother commented, "My brilliant son died of suicide recently. Watching this man's pain helps me on some level. Thank you, dear Ian, for helping me navigate my loss."

The song Paul Simon was composing when he was "crapped out" was "Still Crazy After All These Years," a testament to his unpredictable emotional and mental state. I would certainly add that song to the list.

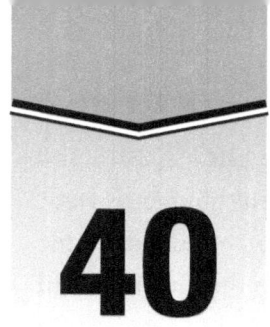

40

Aimee Mann's Masterpiece (Misogyny in Medicine)

"Women who complain about the time they're seen
Sing a different tune when they're on Thorazine."
—Aimee Mann ("Give Me Fifteen")

I've long been a fan of singer songwriter Aimee Mann ("Voices Carry"/'Til Tuesday). Many songs from her 2002 album "Lost in Space" were written around the time she was hospitalized for the treatment of dissociative episodes and PTSD. They could have easily been included in the list of songs mentioned in the previous essay. Mann's songwriting has continued to focus on mental health disorders, stigma, and awareness, including her Grammy Award winning 2018 album titled "Mental Illness" and the 2021 follow-up album, "Queens of the Summer Hotel," which specifically calls out the men of medicine for hastily and incorrectly diagnosing women and labeling them "crazy" simply because they are female.

"Queens of the Summer Hotel" was conceived for a future musical stage adaptation of Susanna Kaysen's 1993 memoir *Girl, Interrupted* – and James Mangold's 1999 Oscar-winning film by the same name – detailing Kaysen's real-life teenage experiences at McLean psychiatric hospital in 1967. The title was inspired by an Anne Sexton poem to her psychiatrist, Dr. Martin T. Orne (1927–2000), who suggested that Sexton begin writing poetry to help unbottle her feelings. Sexton's poem to Orne was written early in her career, after she attempted suicide and while she was a patient at Westwood Lodge psychiatric hospital:

> *"You, Doctor Martin, walk*
> *from breakfast to madness. Late August,*
> *I speed through the antiseptic tunnel*
> *where the moving dead still talk*
> *of pushing their bones against the thrust*
> *of cure. And I am queen of this summer hotel*
> *or the laughing bee on a stalk of death…"*

"I had this idea of calling a mental institution a summer hotel because that just has a lot of weight to it," Mann explained to *SPIN*. Indeed, the therapeutic relationship between Sexton and Orne is considered one of the most intriguing, if not controversial, in the annals of psychiatry. Dr. Orne tape recorded his sessions with Sexton to help compensate for her memory fugues. After Sexton's death, Orne made the tapes available to Sexton's biographer, Dawn M. Skorczewski, without Sexton's explicit permission, drawing the ire of the American Psychiatric Association and others.

Kaysen titled her memoir after a famous baroque painting by the Dutch artist Johannes Vermeer, considered a master of the use of light. The painting is "Girl Interrupted at Her Music" (c. 1660–1). Mann's song, "At the Frick Museum," does not mention the painting by title, but it alludes to the final pages of *Girl, Interrupted,* where 30-something Susanna Kaysen feels drawn to Vermeer's painting, recalling how her life was interrupted 16 years earlier, around the time she first saw the painting (on a high school trip) and prior to her hospitalization at McLean. "At the Frick Museum" recalls:

> *"A strange vignette*
> *In paint and frame*

I knew that, yet
I'd heard my name
Like a dream I'd forgotten
Now it's gone..."

It is noteworthy that the poets Robert Lowell and Sylvia Plath are the subjects of a waltz in "Queens." Along with Sexton and Kaysen, Lowell and Plath were residents at McLean (at different times) and exhibited suicidal tendencies (Plath and Sexton completed suicide). Mood disorders were their defining feature – a gift as well as the source of their suffering – and a common malady among poets and writers (see essay 8). Lowell is famous for saying: "I write when I'm manic and revise when I'm depressed." Mann's song about him and Plath depicts the titular pair walking *"together down the primrose path"* and slowly peels the layers away to detail their downfall:

"Robert Lowell
And Sylvia Plath
Paint and plaster, stripped down
To the lath
One now broken
One now dust
Victim of a
Mental wanderlust..."

Strangely, Lowell mentions a Vermeer painting – most likely "Woman in Blue Reading a Letter" (c.1662–3) – in a poem written toward the end of his career. In the poem, "Epilogue," Lowell compares the writing process to painting – he appears to want to be able to write the way Vermeer paints. Yet, Lowell is self-critical, claiming that sometimes everything he writes seems garish to him. It is known that Lowell especially admires Vermeer's laser focus on people (usually women) completely absorbed in their discipline. Lowell seems to be saying that form and technique are as important in writing as they are in art, and writing poetry is a bright light that gives meaning to his life.

> *"Pray for the grace of accuracy*
> *Vermeer gave to the sun's illumination*
> *stealing like the tide across a map*
> *to his girl solid with yearning.*
> *We are poor passing facts,*
> *warned by that to give*
> *each figure in the photograph*
> *his living name."*

If I had shown more interest in the humanities (essay 14), I would have known about Robert Lowell's distinguished, albeit tortured career and his legacy at my college alma mater, Boston University (BU). In the late 1950s, Lowell led a workshop at BU whose students allegedly included Anne Sexton and Sylvia Plath. This legendary group gathered in a small corner classroom – Room 222 – which is the same room number and title of the 1970s smash television comedy-drama, "Room 222," created by James L. Brooks, whose television and film work includes The Mary Tyler Moore Show, Taxi, The Simpsons, Broadcast News, As Good as It Gets, and Terms of Endearment. I wonder whether Brooks borrowed the title of his hit show from what is now known as the Robert Lowell Seminar Room (222), where today all graduate writing classes and many undergraduate classes at BU are held?

Lowell referenced Boston University in one of his most famous poems, "Walking in the Blue," about his stay at McLean:

> *"The night attendant, a B.U. sophomore,*
> *rouses from the mare's-nest of his drowsy head*
> *propped on The Meaning of Meaning.*
> *He catwalks down our corridor.*

> *Azure day*
> *makes my agonized blue window bleaker.*
> *Crows maunder on the petrified fairway.*
> *Absence! My hearts grows tense*
> *as though a harpoon were sparring for the kill.*
> *(This is the house for the "mentally ill.")…"*

Feminists have written that hysteria epitomized the cult of female invalidism. Nowhere is this more evident than in Mann's song "Give Me Fifteen." She describes a cocky male doctor boasting of his ability to diagnose women in just 15 minutes. How does he do this? Mostly by not really trying to understand women because they "are so simple after all." The brazen doctor prescribes tranquilizers and shock treatment as a 1960s equivalent of hysterectomy. "It's enraging, and every woman has absolutely experienced it – not being taken seriously," Mann told the *Los Angeles Times* (November 4, 2021)

Undoubtedly the most powerful song on "Queens" is "Suicide is Murder." It addresses the repercussion of suicide – loved ones are "cursed, and part of them will also die" – and bespeaks the psychoanalytic notion that behind every suicide there is a homicide. Mann informed *Rolling Stone,* "I started to write this song because I've known people who committed suicide and friends who've had loved ones die from suicide. I think the phrase 'suicide is murder' took on a meaning for me as it's the worst thing to have to deal with in the aftermath. It's just terrible. Because every person who knows the person who committed suicide will blame themselves in some way for not noticing or stepping in or doing something. They'll till the end of their days, say, 'was there something I could have done?'"

Following the heavy lifting, "Queens" ends on a hopeful note: "I See You." The song is a bittersweet denouement encouraging women to battle mental illness and accept support from friends. The narrator of the song reassures a woman that she's not alone: *"There is a girl over a cliff, trying to break her fall – I see you … whether it's black despair or just ennui, I can see."*

In *Girl, Interrupted*, when the "older" Kaysen views Vermeer's paining at the Frick Museum, she sees it differently than she did in high school. Kaysen comments to the girl interrupted at her music – or perhaps to a younger version of herself, or both – "I had something to tell her now. 'I see you.'"

Mann told *Variety* that "I See You" is the song she most identifies with "because that's really about me understanding and acknowledging that there are a lot of people out there who are struggling, and part of the struggle is feeling that people do not understand or will not believe them. Especially if it's PTSD – that's such a huge part of it is to feel like people will believe you."

And so, with "I See You," "Queens" takes one last shot at male doctors – indeed, a plea – to take women's health concerns seriously, especially concerns about mental health, as discussed in essay 29. The message to women is honest and direct: fight for the care you deserve.

If it's any consolation, women today comprise the majority of medical students, and they will surely quash man-made myths about women's bodies and minds once they enter the medical field. In the end, however, it is physicians, those of all persuasions, who must acknowledge and rectify their own biases in order to best serve their patients.

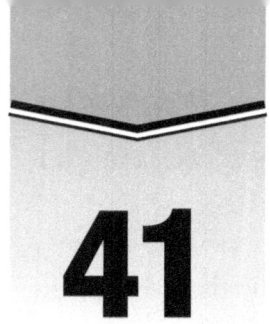

41

Window Shopping on Christmas Eve

Windows are gateways to the human mind.

In 1980, during my first year as a psychiatry resident, I spent a quiet Christmas Eve on call watching "One Flew Over the Cuckoo's Nest" in the day room with about a dozen patients. We all laughed and cried at the same scenes. At that moment, I could not discern any difference between myself and the patients. In Maya Angelou's poem "Human Family," she writes, "In minor ways we differ [but] in major ways we're the same." Collectively, she concludes, "We are more alike, my friends, than we are unalike."

I have been reminded of this certitude countless times in my career, most recently while revisiting the classic 1966 film "Le Roi de Coeur" ("The King of Hearts"), a quirky anti-war fable set in France at the end of World War I. The film's theme and message – who's crazy and who's sane – resemble the motif in Cuckoo's Nest, only the inmates from the asylum have literally escaped and are in command of the town. The colorful patients have a glorious time running the shops before returning to the asylum (Asile D'aliénés), where the last line in the movie is spoken by one of the patients who approaches an open window and exclaims, "The most beautiful journeys are taken through the window."

Peering through windows often gives rise to mental wanderlust – a natural tendency for the mind to wander – from the mundane to fantasy. Random trips into random topics are common and are a form of stress relief. Invariably, windows become fixtures that lead to daydreaming, and although daydreamers have been derided by society, daydreaming is considered a normal and healthy mechanism to overcome old, rusty ways of understanding the world and training the mind to expand even further through introspection and imagination. It is not unusual for a daydream, or series of daydreams, to precede an episode of creative writing or invention. Sometimes the most important revelations and decisions come from looking into a window.

For psychiatric patients confined to mental hospitals, windows provide a way to look at the world outside and imagine the opportunities it offers. The patient Auguste Forestier (1887-1958) was famous for classical wanderlust – the urge to travel widely. His longing for faraway places resulted in repeated escapades around the globe. When he was eventually placed in an asylum and could no longer venture outside, Forestier invented imaginary means of travel and depicted them in his paintings and sculptures, which even Pablo Picasso admired. His wanderlust was unbroken by his detention in a psychiatric facility, prompting his psychiatrist to comment: "Forestier's work will always bear traces of the ideal of the traveler."

What happens to the human mind when travel is prevented or restricted, as with all types of institutional confinement, including incarceration, and during epidemics such as COVID-19? Here, I rely on my clinical experience and recall my first encounter with a psychiatric patient. In my third year of medical school, I was assigned to a state-run mental institution for my psychiatry clerkship. I approached the locked psychiatric ward with trepidation and skeleton key in hand. The key was provided to open the locked door to the inpatient unit. "The only way you can flunk this rotation," my attending said, "is to lose the key."

A tiny woman was peering through the window of the corridor door separating us. She had been awaiting my arrival. I inserted the key, and as I turned it, the woman backed away and dashed into her room. Slowly opening the door, I entered the ward. I quickly turned around to relock it. Suddenly, the woman sprang from the doorway of her room and fixed her gaze on me. "Hey, Mr. DJ," she shouted, "are you the postman?"

Those were the first words uttered to me by a psychiatric patient. I should have considered another medical specialty from the outset. But the absurdity of this patient's comment intrigued me. Her remark unmasked a profoundly disturbed and psychotic woman, and her question clearly indicated a longing for contact with the outside world. She wanted someone to correspond with her. She wanted mail.

Windows have symbolic meanings in psychiatry. Peering through them may reveal opportunity, desire, and yearning. Windows also symbolize liberation. Recall that in the final scene of "Cuckoo's Nest," Chief Bromden finally has the courage to break free from the hospital. He escapes through a window after smashing it the way McMurphy had told him to – by grabbing a huge bathroom sink and plucking it from its base. As the other patients look on in shock, the Chief leaps through the window and into the open field. He has regained his freedom.

Although windows provide welcome light from the outside, they also may pose a threat by virtue of what the light might show, e.g., character flaws or other pathology prime for psychoanalysis. Psychotherapy is an ambivalent, uncomfortable experience for many patients. Their reluctance to open a window – "open up" in therapy (or as a writer [essay 3]) – is one reason many sessions often are required before any improvement is seen.

Windows are a compelling metaphor to capture psychiatrists' efforts to create access to the inner world of their patients. The phrase "windows to the unconscious" was coined by Sigmund Freud to label techniques for diagnosing hidden problems, such as dream interpretation. Tinted windows may shield patients from real or perceived threats in the environment. They must become translucent in order for psychoanalysis to proceed successfully.

Windows often separate observers from participants. For example, individuals who tend to be isolated and disconnected from society commonly enjoy a rich inner life, but they are not fully engaged with their peers or with social activities. Windows represent a visual bridge between the interior and the exterior, filtering elements that may frighten some yet entice others. The frightened stay behind while the adventurous cross over and seek new experiences. It's no wonder that today's wanderers speak of self-discovery and wanting to lose themselves to accomplish internal change. Without internal change, they argue, there is no fulfillment or meaning in life.

Although many individuals stare out of windows, in certain instances windows are feared. Some people only feel safe when inside their homes; they dread going out, especially in crowded or public spaces (agoraphobia). The plane of glass shields them physically; however, they are exposed psychologically and are vulnerable to the chaos of the external environment. For those individuals, windows represent something to avoid – except when the temptation to stare or gawk overrides their fear, as in Alfred Hitchcock's "Rear Window." The voyeur L.B. Jeffries ("Jeff," played by Jimmy Stewart) would rather look at the lives of others through a window, aided by a telephoto lens on his camera, than live inside his own skin.

Windows may hold special meaning for physicians by connecting their hobbies to their specialties and by influencing how physicians spend their free time. When general surgeon Steven Immerman, MD, recognized he needed a hobby that would allow him to work with his hands, he turned to kiln-formed glass art. Immerman attended a workshop and proposed a project – a block of colored glass with a window through which viewers could observe the contents inside – and the instructor remarked, "Well, of course. You're a surgeon. You make little openings in people and you look inside."

Painters, poets, and musicians have added depth to the symbolism of windows in psychiatry. Joni Mitchell has described life *"from both sides . . . from up and down . . . from win and lose."* I mentioned the Dutch baroque artist Johannes Vermeer in the previous essay. His paintings famously reflected light streaming through windows. I also discussed singer-songwriter Aimee Mann and the "confessional" poets Sylvia Plath, Anne Sexton, and Robert Lowell. These artists and innumerable others have incorporated psychological dimensions of storytelling and affirmation in their works, illuminated through a window of creative expression.

Windows are gateways to the human mind, and looking through them is a time-honored exercise in reflection and introspection. Although people appear to be looking outward, they are really looking within to find answers or explore new possibilities and terrain. Sometimes, when I stare out the window and daydream, I see myself in the window's reflection, at first blurred, then gradually coming into focus. It's a reminder that there's a thin line between sane and insane, between normal and crazy. I feel humbled. I'm transported back to the psychiatry day room watching "Cuckoo's Nest" on the television. I'm in the company of patients who are psychiatrically ill yet acting normal. They are my family on Christmas Eve. They are more like me than unalike.

AFTERWORD

42

Should You Publish Your Narrative?

Telling your story may be powerful enough.

I don't like being rejected. Who does? But I got a real chuckle once when I received a rejection letter from an editor affiliated with a prominent website, a repository for doctors' essays and op-eds. The letter read:

"Thanks for your submission. It looks like you have another article about narrative medicine already in the pipeline to be published, and we don't want to oversaturate that subject, especially by the same author. We will pass on publication of this piece, but welcome you to subject (sic) other works, especially if they are not on narrative medicine."

Here's the punchline: the title of the article was "Why Aren't You Writing?" (essay 4, which I eventually published elsewhere). It was an essay written to encourage physicians to write expressively about their encounters – with patients, peers, trainees – anything to take their mind off the drudgery of everyday practice and to help them reduce stress. Do you see the humor here? An essay about writing, suited for a website that invites written commentary from physicians, was rejected precisely because the essay was about writing!

Furthermore, the letter was unsigned, and I suspect that the editor made a major Freudian slip when they wrote "subject" instead of "submit." Was I "subjecting" the editor to a narrative so unpleasant that they did not even want to attach their name to the rejection letter? Did I torture the editor by writing about the need for more narratives in the medical profession?

I hope not.

This brings me to the main message I want to leave with readers: write, write, write. And then write some more. There were many subjects I wanted to tackle in writing this book, but the chief objective was to encourage physicians – indeed, anyone remotely connected to health care – to write. Write for nourishment. Write for your patients. Write for any reason you want to write. Capture your thoughts in a journal and write later if you don't have the time now.

And don't be afraid of rejection.

Most of you have heard the famous Michael Jordan quote about failure. It's so good, I want you to read it again, or perhaps for the first time:

"I've lost almost 300 games. Twenty-six times, I've been trusted to take the game winning shot and missed. I've failed over and over and over again in my life. And that is why I succeed."

I've lost count of the number of times my writing has been rejected for publication. Several times I've thought my essays were the right stuff for *JAMA*'s column "A Piece of My Mind," a column "devoted to telling stories about the joys, challenges, and hidden truths of practicing medicine in the modern era." I have been reading that column for a long time and I admire those successful *JAMA* authors whose narratives are chosen for publication. I want to be one of them.

Certainly not everything I've written is *JAMA* quality, but some essays I do believe were good candidates. Over the past five years I have submitted no less than a dozen essays to *JAMA* for consideration in "A Piece of My Mind," and every one of them has been rejected, all with the same form letter:

> "Dear Dr Lazarus:
>
> We have now completed our review of your manuscript. I am sorry to inform you that we will not be able to publish the manuscript.
>
> Every year we receive hundreds of manuscripts. Criteria for determining acceptance include priority, originality, quality, and appeal for our general medical audience. Unfortunately, your manuscript was judged by the editors not to have met the criteria necessary for publication in *JAMA*.
>
> We were pleased to have had the opportunity to review your work. Thank you for thinking of *JAMA*.
>
> Sincerely yours,
> Deputy Editor"

Letters like these won't deter me from writing. I'll keep at it and try to publish my essays somewhere else. I'll find a home for them somewhere, even if I have to publish them myself on *Medium*, bypassing editors. My strong will and inner drive to publish articles led medical students and residents to call me "Article" Lazarus (essay 22), and I achieved much publication success throughout my career. Rejection does not come easy for me.

I've been told I'm "rejection sensitive." I wouldn't argue that characterization. Decades ago, psychiatrists diagnosed some people with "rejection-sensitive dysphoria." Psychiatrists no longer use that term in an official capacity, but the possibility is raised by having several of the characteristics below:

- High sensitivity about the possibility of rejection

- Overly high standards for yourself
- Feeling easily triggered toward guilt or shame
- Isolating yourself in a preemptive strike not to be rejected
- Aggressive or rageful behavior toward those who have been perceived to have slighted you
- Frequently feeling an uncomfortable physical reaction due to "not fitting in" or being misunderstood
- Self-esteem that is entirely dependent on what others think, and rises and falls accordingly
- Frequent and intense ruminating after an interaction about how you did or said something wrong

As my career progressed, I found that taking things easier and ridding myself of publication envy tempered my reaction to editors who rejected my manuscripts. It may sound counter to all I have said so far, but I don't want to leave you with the impression that publication is the main goal of writing narratives – it's not! It's nice to publish, but it's not critical or even desirable in some instances.

Nearly a dozen essays in this book were never submitted for publication because, as Doximity intimated, I did not want to "saturate" my usual sources, my go-to websites, with essays about the virtues of writing narratives. I saved them for this book, which I self-published. If you're writing for yourself, for your own therapy, to enhance your well-being, to inform patients, to educate the public, then publication is secondary. There are ways to share your written work besides formally publishing it, e.g., through social media and various mediums of storytelling.

I would encourage you to get more involved in storytelling. Danish author Isak Dinesen (Karen Blixen), author of *Out of Africa* and other novels, remarked: "To be a person is to have a story to tell." Yet stories haven't received the credit they deserve as a legitimate path to healing. Telling stories helps us heal as we wind our way through illness, trauma, and loss. Stories help us reframe our struggles, and they can transform our lives and the lives of others. There is no doubt stories are powerful.

Putting them on paper is key.

Publishing them is optional.

Notes and Sources

Many essays in this book were posted online in 2023 at one of several websites: KevinMD, MedPage Today and Doximity. They were edited and cross-referenced during the book's production. References to medical research, scientific studies, and quotations were intentionally omitted in order to improve the continuity of reading. To access source information, readers can search the essays by their titles on the Internet and click on hyperlinked text embedded within each essay.

Essay 17 was adapted with permission from *The Physician Leadership Journal* 2015, Volume 2 Number 5, pages 68-70, American Association for Physician Leadership®, 800-562-8088, www.physicianleaders.org

Essays 36 and 37 were adapted with permission from *The Journal of Medical Practice Management* 2020, Volume 35 Number 5, pages 266-269, American Association for Physician Leadership®, 800-562-8088, www.physicianleaders.org

Essay 38 was adapted with permission from *The Journal of Medical Practice Management* 2019, Volume 35 Number 1, pages 47-50, American Association for Physician Leadership®, 800-562-8088, www.physicianleaders.org

Essay 41 was adapted with permission from *The Journal of Medical Practice Management* 2022, Volume 37 Number 6, pages 295-297, American Association for Physician Leadership®, 800-562-8088, www.physicianleaders.org